BASIC PSYCHIATRY

BASIC PSYCHIATRY

MYRE SIM

M.D.(Edin), F.R.C.P.(Edin), F.R.C.Psych., F.R.C.P.(C), D.P.M.

Professor of Psychiatry, Faculty of Medicine, University of Ottawa, Ontario,
Canada; formerly Consultant Psychiatrist, United Birmingham Hospitals

E. B. GORDON

M.B., Ch.B.(Edin), M.R.C.Psych., D.P.M.

Consultant Psychiatrist, Saxondale Hospital and General Hospital, Nottingham
Postgraduate Clinical Tutor, University of Sheffield
Clinical Teacher to the University of Nottingham

THIRD EDITION

CHURCHILL LIVINGSTONE
EDINBURGH LONDON AND NEW YORK
1976

CHURCHILL LIVINGSTONE

Medical Division of Longman Group Limited

Distributed in the United States of America by
Longman Inc., 19 West 44th street, New York,
N.Y. 10036 and by associated companies,
branches and representatives throughout
the world.

First Edition 1968
Second Edition 1972
  Reprinted 1974
Third Edition 1976

ISBN 0 443 01341 1

Library of Congress Cataloging in Publication Data

Sim, Myre.
  Basic psychiatry.

  Includes index.
  1. Psychiatry. I. Gordon, Edward Benjamin, joint
author. II. Title. [DNLM: 1. Mental disorders. WM100
S589b]
RC454.S46   1976   616.8′9   75-38609

Reproduced, printed and bound in Great Britain by
Morrison & Gibb Ltd, London and Edinburgh

PREFACE TO THE THIRD EDITION

This book continues to gain in popularity, not only in English-speaking countries, for there is now an Italian translation. Fresh editions add to the responsibilities of authors who have to ensure that only essential new material is included, and what is even more difficult, that inessential old material is excluded. This we have tried to do and we hope that our readers will find this edition no less useful than its predecessors.

M. S.
E. G.

Ottawa, Ontario, Canada.
Nottingham, England.
1976

PREFACE TO THE SECOND EDITION

The success of the First Edition would indicate that the need declared by our own students for a short textbook of psychiatry which uses the question and answer method and which briefly summarizes the essential data is shared by many others. A common criticism by reviewers, though less so by students, was the absence of an alphabetical index. We have now included one, though we still retain the extended Table of Contents, each item of which represents a question and answer complex.

All Sections have been updated and omissions from the First Edition have been remedied. It was possible to do some pruning, so the book has not grown materially and we hope it will be even more useful than its predecessor.

1971   MYRE SIM
                                                       E. B. GORDON

PREFACE TO THE FIRST EDITION

Psychiatry is now a required subject, not only for medical students but for nurses, occupational therapists, social workers, psychologists and others. Many students have expressed their need for a book which would deal with the subject in the manner we generally adopt in our teaching; that of question and answer. This, they say, highlights the relevance of information to the type of problem they may expect to meet in their professional work and in examinations.

This form of presentation appeals to those who wish to gain from a small volume a ready understanding of the basic aspects of the subject and at the same time get the help they need in formulating answers. There are others who, in addition to a larger text, require a small book for rapid revision. In response to these requests we have tried to reproduce our teaching in book form.

We have dispensed with the customary alphabetical index and substituted a full Table of Contents. This should prove more convenient for the type of reader we envisage.

1968   MYRE SIM
                                                       E. B. GORDON

TABLE OF CONTENTS

SECTION 1

PSYCHOLOGY

What are **motives** *and how are they classified?*

A *motive* is something that incites the organism to activity or sustains and gives direction to activity, after the organism has been aroused. Motives thus have activating as well as directing aspects.

Classification. Any classification of motives must be arbitrary, since some motives seem to be primary, whereas others are expressed through learned behaviour. Again, the learned motives are usually influenced by environmental factors, e.g. family and socio-cultural milieu. Motives may occur in distorted or disguised forms and any one pattern of behaviour may be influenced by several motives.

(a) *Survival motives*

This group is closely related to bodily needs, e.g. food, water, elimination, etc., therefore hunger and thirst are included. Survival motives, referred to as *drives*, include finding optimum levels of activity and rest, escaping from pain and danger, and the satisfaction of curiosity.

(b) *Social motives*

These involve dealing with other individuals and groups and may influence the survival of the species, through sex and parenthood. They also include dependency needs and needs for affiliation to the group, as is observed at family, society, subcultural and national levels. Anxiety, or any threatening situation, increases these needs in most individuals.

Dominance and submission are motives which are also seen at a social level in most species, e.g. pecking order in hens, human ranks and hierarchy.

Aggression is often regarded as being due to the frustration of

1

motivated behaviour, but according to psychoanalytic theory, aggression (like sex) is regarded as a primary need or drive.

(c) *Ego-integrative motives*

These refer to the 'self'; and apply to such motives as achieving one's aims or goals, leading to attempts at mastery of the environment. The achievement motive, like the other ego-integrative motives, is largely based on earlier learning experiences, and it has been demonstrated that the achievement-orientation of the particular culture is an important factor.

It has been generally accepted since Freud that many motives are unconscious, or partly unconscious, in nature.

Describe the theory of **motivation**

1. *The need-drive theory*

Bodily needs give rise to drives, i.e. physiological deficiencies produce psychological motivation. The drive thus produced leads to goal-directed behaviour. For example, food depletion leads to the hunger drive, with consequent food seeking as the goal. When the goal is reached, the hunger drive is reduced. Drive-reduction has been proposed as one basis for the function of rewards in enhancing learning.

Some suggest there is one drive, e.g. any active drive contributes to a general state of activity. Others favour the multiple-drive interpretation, e.g. appetitive-drives, such as the seeking of food, are distinguished from aversive drives such as the avoidance of pain.

2. *The cue-stimulus (non-drive) theory*

Behaviour is a response to a stimulus and when stimulus conditions are appropriate, the relevant habit is brought into action.

3. *Affective arousal*

Emotional responses are held to determine motivated behaviour. The expectation of pleasure or pain, based on previous experience, is said to 'control motivated action'. This theory postulates that emotional consequences are important features of motivated behaviour; that an aspect of goal-seeking in appetitive motives is pleasure, and an aspect of avoidance behaviour is pain or discomfort.

4. *Cognitive theories*

It is implied that some form of choice or understanding is exercised which is based on previous experience, present circumstances or future predictions. Factors included in such theories are levels of aspiration, value of incentives and rewards and consideration of risks involved.

5. *Psychoanalytic theory*

Sex and aggression are regarded as the basic or primitive drives and these undergo various object attachments during the stages of psychosexual development. Ego defence mechanisms help to deal with the activity and direction of drives. (See Section 2.)

What are **instincts?**

Instinct is defined as unlearned, patterned, goal-directed behaviour which is species-specific. Examples include nest-building in birds, migration of salmon, and the behaviour of the larva of the Capricorn beetle. Instincts are often referred to as 'species-specific behaviour' or 'innate responses'. Although instincts are supposed to be unlearned, they are influenced by factors such as maturation and practice.

William James suggested that man was more richly endowed with instincts than any other animal, and added that these were transient and became replaced by habit systems. McDougall later proposed a theory of human instincts which became the central theme of his system of psychology in which he included 18 groups. Much of this earlier work on human instinct neglected the fact that acquired habits could themselves act as drives. A major disagreement between earlier theories of instinct was this inconstant use of the term.

The term is now reserved for certain types of behaviour among the *lower animals*, characterised by automatic and invariable innate responses.

What were previously regarded as *human* instincts now fall into the following categories:

1. Drive, based on physiological needs.
2. Motives, which may be elaborate and based on learning.
3. Maturational development, e.g. some behaviour characteristics of a baby.

Early instinct theory is of historical importance, since it constituted the first break from the old associationist psychology which had failed to provide an understanding of human behaviour.

What is meant by **imprinting**?

Spalding's early experiments with chicks demonstrated the tendency of young birds to accept the first suitable moving object which presents itself for the reaction of following. Lorenz, and others of the school of *ethology*, confirmed these findings and named this process, whereby an instinctive reaction becomes specific to the object which happens to be present at the time the organism is ready to adopt a specific object, *imprinting*. The process depends on there being a critical time during which the learning occurs and its effects are not reversible. Examples in animals include the reaction of following in birds, and the acquisition by chaffinches of their species-specific song. It is unlikely that the process of imprinting has any human applications, though there is a psychologist-ethnologist trend of thought which postulates that it may be analogous to the development of emotional attachments to particular objects.

What are the various modes of **learning**?

1. Classical conditioning.
2. Operant conditioning.
3. Multiple-response learning.
4. 'Learning with understanding'.

Describe the principles underlying **classical conditioning**

In classical conditioning, a stimulus which already has the power to elicit a response is presented in contiguity with another stimulus which does not yet have this ability. Repetition of the presentation of these two stimuli ultimately leads to the previously neutral stimulus eliciting the response when it is presented on its own. The stimulus which originally elicits the response is the *unconditioned stimulus* and the response, the *unconditioned response*. The previously neutral stimulus is the *conditioned stimulus* and the response, when made to that stimulus alone, the *conditioned response*.

Reinforcement refers to the contiguous presentation of a conditioned stimulus and an unconditioned stimulus. Conditioned responses to the conditioned stimulus appear consequently at progressively greater strength and with greater regularity as the paired stimulation is repeated.

Once formed, the conditioned response undergoes changes in strength. Repetition of the conditioned stimulus without reinforcement is called *extinction*. It has been shown that decrease in response during extinction is not merely a disappearance of the response but is an active process of *inhibition*. The latter process may in fact spread to other responses not originally included in the conditioning. Following a period of rest, the conditioned response reappears, even without any reinforcement having taken place, through the process of *spontaneous recovery*.

Generalisation refers to the phenomenon whereby stimuli similar to the original stimulus producing the conditioned response can also evoke the response, e.g. in the type of experiment originally carried out by Pavlov on dogs, the animal may learn to salivate to the sound of a tuning fork; generalisation allows salivation to take place also in response to tuning forks of different tones. Generalisation is important in learning, since it enables the individual to react to new situations, on the basis of their similarities to familiar ones.

Discrimination is analogous to generalisation, in that differences, as opposed to similarities, are reacted to; in this way, conditioned discrimination between two conditioned stimuli can occur.

Avoidance learning refers to the establishment of *avoidance responses*. To establish the latter, a conditioned stimulus is paired with a painful unconditioned stimulus, e.g. a painful electric shock, in circumstances whereby the subject can avoid receiving the shock provided that he makes a premeditated response when the conditioned stimulus appears. The response is said to be learned when the subject is able to avoid the shock a significantly large number of times.

It is hypothesised that some acquired fears or phobias in patients occur in accordance with principles of classical conditioning, the conditioned avoidance response being a commonly employed mechanism. In such situations, the feared danger acts as the unconditioned stimulus.

What is meant by **operant conditioning?**

Operant conditioning, also called instrumental behaviour, refers to the strengthening of a stimulus-response association by following the response with a reinforcing stimulus. Experimental models of this type of learning can be constructed by means of the 'Skinner box'. A hungry rat is placed in the box and will move about aimlessly, occasionally pressing a bar. If food is liberated every time the bar is pressed, the rat presses the bar with greater frequency, i.e. the food acts as a reinforcing stimulus.

The learning that takes place in operant conditioning corresponds to classical conditioning with regard to the principles of extinction (no reinforcement), spontaneous recovery, generalisation and discrimination (selective reinforcement, e.g. presenting food only if the bar is pressed while a light is on). The phenomenon of secondary reinforcement occurs in classical conditioning, but more readily in operant conditioning. The principle is that any stimulus can be made reinforcing through association with a reinforcing stimulus. In the well-known chimpanzee experiments, the animals learned to exert considerable effort to obtain grapes, but subsequently also to acquire poker chips which could be exchanged for grapes. The importance of secondary reinforcement is that it enables a wide margin of generalisation to occur, thus subjecting a wide range of behaviour to the influence of secondary reinforcers. It is thought that social approval can act as a powerful secondary reinforcer.

The principles of operant conditioning have been applied to various clinical problems. For example, hysterical blindness was treated successfully by rewarding the patient with tokens when presentation of light provoked the pressing of a lever.

The rewarding of patients with tokens which can later be exchanged for various items has been used to reinforce various types of desirable behaviour and habits in chronic schizophrenics and subnormals. It is called *token economy treatment*.

What is multiple-response learning?

This type of learning is far more complex than conditioning, although both forms are probably responsible for many types of habit formation. Conditioning applies to single, identifiable responses, whereas multiple-response learning includes more than one identifiable act.

Examples:

1. Maze learning.
2. Mirror-drawing experiments, in which the subject has to trace a path round a figure while viewing it in a mirror.
3. Rote memorisation. The pioneer study in this field was by Ebbinghaus, who employed nonsense syllables.

Multiple-response learning can be quantified (e.g. number of trials against scores) and the results plotted to form a *learning curve*. Such a curve indicates changes in proficiency with practice; it usually shows decreasing gains per trial. It is possible that the S-shaped curve is the commonest form for overall learning; the S-shape shows increasing gains at first, with subsequent decreasing gains.

Describe the forms of learning *not attributable to conditioning*

Non-conditioning types of learning are often referred to as 'learning with understanding' or 'learning with insight'.

Köhler was the first to demonstrate in the psychological laboratory a type of learning which did not depend on conditioning. Chimpanzees were able to obtain food outside a cage by employing sticks. The animals seemed to grasp the essentials of the problem to be solved, i.e. they had *insight,* and did not merely arrive ultimately at the solution by trial and error. Much of human learning involves achieving insight, which depends on various factors, including innate ability to learn from an appropriate previous experience. Köhler's experiments showed how the arrangements of the problem determine the relative ease of solution, and how a solution once achieved with insight, no matter how sudden, can be repeated or applied to new situations.

Sign learning is another form of learning which is said to be not attributable to conditioning. Tolman hypothesised that much learning is sign learning, e.g. an experimental animal may be able to run through a maze by learning a map of the maze. This form of learning involves the knowledge that one stimulus will be followed by another, provided that certain behaviour is undertaken. It proposes that the organism learns the location of certain routes and sign-posts instead of learning habits of movement.

What are the main stages of **memory?**

1. *Acquisition*

The first stage in remembering involves previous *learning* of data which can be retained. Learning is enhanced by good motivation and also depends on attention at the time of learning. There are various types of learning, e.g. by conditioning, reward, multiple-response learning including rote learning, and learning with understanding. The type of learning is not as important for the psychological process of remembering as the degree to which the learned material is *retained*. Recent research has pointed to various factors which may be of importance in the matter of retention. An example is the sequences in which the material for learning is presented. There is evidence that learned material is retained through a process of encoding, i.e. the information learned is coded in one of several ways, e.g. by employing words having some particular quality or those occurring frequently in normal language.

Relearning a particular task is usually quicker than the first attempt at learning, since there has been some retention of previously learned material.

2. *Storage*

Learned data must be stored; there is neurophysiological evidence that DNA and long-tract neuronal pathways in the brain may be concerned, but the psychological basis of storage is still uncertain. In the past, the 'memory trace' has been regarded as the inferred physical basis of memory.

3. *Retrieval*

The final stage in remembering involves the recognition and recall of information or experiences.

Recognition implies that something, or someone, strikes one as being familiar, i.e. has been associated with a previous experience, and therefore with some old 'memory trace'. Recognition can be studied in the psychological laboratory by testing a subject's ability to distinguish between correct and faulty recognition, e.g. using photographs.

Recall implies the active recollection of some performance learned previously. This is easily tested in the laboratory, employing words, sequences of words, objects, etc. Ability to recall previously learned material is bound up with ability to recognise the latter or parts of the latter as being familiar. In retrieval, the processes of recognition and recall are employed and it has been shown in the psychological laboratory that some of the clues and short-hand methods that are used initially come into play in the stage of acquisition, i.e. in the earlier processes of learning and retention. Such techniques include classifying links between words, linking certain facts together, and other coding methods.

What is meant by **redintegration**?

This term, used by psychologists, refers to remembering the whole of an earlier experience on the basis of partial ones, and is usually concerned with events and relevant circumstances in the individual's personal history. This aspect of memory has often been investigated under hypnosis and in psychotherapy in an attempt to reactivate early experiences.

Describe the theories of **forgetting**

1. *Dynamic*

This postulates that forgetting occurs on the basis of *repression* i.e. emotionally toned facts and experiences are repressed from the conscious mind into the unconscious. It is true that everyone represses certain events in their life but repression certainly cannot account for all forgetting. This theory is often referred to as 'motivated forgetting'.

2. *Passive decay through disuse*

This theory suggests that forgetting is due to fading or decay of 'memory traces' in the brain, with the passage of time. The experience of rapid fading of recently learned, or poorly learned material is a common one, as is the forgetting of jokes, stories, etc.

One argument against this theory is the fact that senile patients may remember far-off events, but not recent ones.

3. *Distortion of the memory trace*

Early recollection of events frequently differs from later recollections. This theory suggests that forgetting occurs through distortion of events, by means of systematic distortion of the memory trace. This distortion is said to be caused by spontaneous changes in the memory trace, and does not seem to be related to the passage of time. Experiments that test this theory include different witnesses giving testimony to the same event and the reproduction of various figures and designs.

4. *Inhibition*

This implies that retention of old material is interfered with through the acquisition of new information ('retroactive inhibition'). A similar theory, also implicating inhibition, involves 'proactive inhibition', i.e. prior learning can also interfere with the acquisition and retrieval of new material. One of the facts supporting the theory of retroactive inhibition is the greater likelihood of forgetting learned material after some hours' waking activity than after a similar interval of sleep.

Discuss the 'associationist' schools of psychology

The earlier psychologists frequently examined the ability of individuals to recall information by enquiring, in retrospect, about the associations in the conscious mind, and by examining the processes through which these associations were made. In later 'associationist' schools, the process of forming associations was the starting-point, and the strength of these associations were subsequently tested by recall. *Ebbinghaus* performed pioneer experiments by investigating the associations formed in learning and the variables which influenced the learning process, e.g. mode and speed of learning, mental activity in the interval between learning, and later recall. To achieve objectivity he invented nonsense syllables for use in his investigations.

Studies on learning in dogs led to different interpretations, e.g.

that the learning process involved the formation of simple associations (Wundt) or that dogs learned by trial and error (Lloyd
Morgan). Higher mental processes were not thought to play any
part in learning.

Further research led to new laws of association. *Thorndike's*
experiments on learning in various animals, especially the cat, led
to his *'law of effect'* which stated that any act which produces
satisfaction in a given situation becomes associated with that
situation. His accompanying *law of exercise* inferred the formation
of similar associations, but between situation and response and not
between ideas. *Pavlov*, performing conditioning experiments on
dogs, enunciated his *laws of reinforcement*, the latter referring to
the contiguous presentation of a conditioned stimulus and an
unconditioned stimulus, and the progressive strengthening of the
conditioned response with repeated paired stimulation. Later,
the closeness of Thorndike's laws and Pavlov's principles of
conditioning was acknowledged. The gap between these theories
was bridged by *Skinner*, whose classical experiments employing the 'Skinner box', demonstrated the role of reward in
'reinforced learning'. His 'instrumental learning' is in fact the
same process as Pavlov's 'operant conditioning' (which implies
reinforcement), and implicates the same principles as Thorndike's
'reward'.

Common to all the associationist schools of psychology is the
theme of the importance of links, i.e. associations, in any theory of
learning and remembering.

Write a note on **Wundt**

Wilhelm Wundt was one of the originators of the group of
psychological theories often called *'associationist'*. He believed
that conscious experience constituted the main subject of study of
psychology, and that discovering the elements of conscious experience should be the primary aim. His brand of psychology was
often referred to as *'structural psychology'*. He postulated that all
experiences, e.g. perceptions of external objects, emotions and
memories had a rather complex structure that called for scientific
analysis. Wundt suggested that experiences could be analysed
and divided into two main groups: (i) sensations arising in the
environment and (ii) feelings belonging to the individual; the

sensations and feelings were accordingly subdivided. He proposed various laws, according to which the elements of experience could combine and blend in various patterns and combinations. One such law is his *'principle of creative synthesis'*, which states that combination creates new properties. Wundt distinguished between *perception* and *apperception*, the latter being a special form of perception, where attention is directly paid to the sensory stimulus which is being perceived.

He laid the foundations of experimentation in psychological laboratories, and his ideas influenced early psychiatry, e.g. the clinical use of word-association tests and Bleuler's views on thought disorder.

Discuss behaviourism

The founder of Behaviourism was *Watson*, who objected to the study of conscious experience by introspection. He believed that the reactions of men and animals could be better examined by means of objective measure, e.g. physiological secretions, movements, etc.

His views included the following:

1. *Behaviour* can be analysed in terms of simple stimulus-response units which he termed reflexes. This was the forerunner of modern 'stimulus-response' (S-R) psychology, where the emphasis is placed on describing psychological events as beginning with a stimulus and ending with a response.
2. *Thinking* is based on implicit muscle responses, and can be reduced to sensorimotor activity.
3. *Emotion.* Only the stimuli in the situation, the accompanying response and the relevant visceral changes are important; any conscious concomitant of emotion is denied.
4. *Learning.* Law of exercise and conditioning are the only important factors.
5. *Instinct and heredity* of mental attributes do not exist.

Lashley, a pupil of Watson, is often regarded as belonging to the behaviourist school, although most of his research has been directed to the effect of brain lesions on learning, e.g. cortex destruction and maze learning in rats. He enunciated two principles:

1. Principle of equipotentiality: one part of the cortex is potentially the same as another in its capacity for learning. Notable exception is the visual area.

2. Principle of mass action: the more cortex remaining, the more effective the learning.

In general, Lashley's work rejects the theories of the earlier behaviourists who were ready to attribute brain function and learning to simple reflexes.

Later behaviourists include Tolman, Clark Hull and Skinner.

Tolman rebelled against Watson's denial of introspection and purpose, and pointed out that even a rat's trial-and-error behaviour in a maze is goal directed and purposive. He postulated that between the environmental stimulus and the response of the animal lie many 'intervening variables', some of which are cognitive, while others refer to demands for sex, safety, etc.

Clark Hull's views are as much 'modern associationist' as they are behaviourist. His central theme is the stimulus-response association, but with emphasis on drive, which is equivalent to one of Tolman's intervening variables. Hull applied principles of Pavlovian conditioning, and used such terms as reinforcement and extinction. He postulated that any stimulus which is closely approximated in time to a reinforced response becomes associated with that response so as to evoke it later. He has made a strong impact on the psychology of motives and drives, particularly with his suggestion that reduction of a need or drive is important in reinforcement of learning.

Skinner adheres to the traditional behaviourist view that behaviour is composed of reflexes which are basically stimulus-response units but he emphasises the variables in the experimental situation. He developed the Skinner puzzle box for rat experiments, and his results do seem to bridge the gap between Pavlov's conditioning and Thorndike's trial and error. Skinner postulates 'operant reflexes' which operate on the environment and in fact are instrumental, e.g. rats' approach to the food; and instrumental behaviour which is instrumental in obtaining the reward which reinforces. Skinner suggests that a long series of stimulus-response units can be elaborated by appropriate conditioning, thus leading to a more complex pattern of behaviour. His work has had, and still maintains, a powerful influence on modern psychological theory.

Give a brief outline of Gestalt psychology

The beginnings of Gestalt psychology are associated with the names of Wertheimer, Koffka and Köhler. The original experiments dealt with perceived motion, e.g. in viewing a motion picture. The first principle in this school of psychology soon became apparent, viz. that a whole was not merely a sum of parts. Other experiments concerned 'figure-and-ground', i.e. a tendency to see part of a pattern as an object in the foreground against an unstructured background. Thus, attention was paid to the background of an object as well as to the shape of the object, and 'Gestalt' means shape. According to Gestalt psychologists, our experiences depend on the patterns formed by stimuli and on the organisation of our perceptual field. The Austrian Gestalt school postulated that a higher mental process was responsible for the organisation of sensations. The Berlin school (Wertheimer, Koffka, and Köhler) believed that there were general factors involved in the process of organisation: (i) peripheral factors, in the stimuli, e.g. proximity, similarity and closure; (ii) central factors, originating in the organism, e.g. familiarity, set, attitude; (iii) reinforcing factors, analogous to the reinforcement of a conditioned response.

Later developments in Gestalt psychology regarded mental processes as dynamic, often employing the 'field concept' and an analogy with field theory in physics. They felt that not only sensory experiences but behaviour in general demonstrated wholes which were not merely sums of parts; and that a close relationship existed between seen or heard patterns and the corresponding brain processes. Koffka postulated that behaviour was governed by a field, the organismic field of interacting forces. Such forces tended to be in equilibrium, including the 'Gestalten'.

Gestalt psychology also includes the work of Köhler with apes, demonstrating that these animals could learn with *insight* or understanding, as opposed to simpler forms of learning. It was demonstrated that insight was associated with (i) the sudden transformation from helplessness to mastery of a problem; (ii) good retention of the learned phenomenon and (iii) transfer of learning to similar tasks.

Field theory, the main proponent being Kurt Lewin, is a variant of Gestalt psychology. Although psychological forces are postulated, they are related not to physical forces in the environment nor to brain dynamics, but to social factors. Lewin's field is the 'life space, containing the person and his psychological environment'. Field theory is in fact very much concerned with social behaviour and motivation. Mathematical symbols, including vector analysis to represent motives, are employed to construct experimental models to test hypotheses. Tensions in various human situations are thus explored and analysed.

What psychological tests are commonly used in the **assessment of intelligence?**

1. *Stanford-Binet Scale*

Used primarily for children. For the testing of young children (2 years +), various sub-tests are available, employing manipulation of blocks, beads, drawing and copying. For the older child, there are scales which measure arithmetical ability, discrimination and recognition of patterns, picture completion, similarities and differences between objects. In the upper age-ranges, verbal tests become more prominent. The use of this scale enables an I.Q. to be estimated.

2. *Group Intelligence Tests*

Many tests are available which can be given to a group of people simultaneously. Raven's Progressive Matrices is a popular example. It was designed to measure Spearman's 'g' factor, and is completely non-verbal, therefore the results do not depend on education. The test consists of 60 matrices or abstract designs grouped in five sets of 12. Each design has a missing part, and the candidate selects the latter from a group of six or eight represented below. There is an alternative 'Matrices' which employs coloured designs which can be used for children or deteriorated adults.

The Mill Hill Vocabulary Scale is linked with Raven's Matrices and measures verbal ability.

3. *Wechsler Adult Intelligence Scale* (WAIS)

This is the most commonly used test of adult intelligence,

initially being presented as the Wechsler-Bellevue Scale. There are two sections:

(a) *Verbal Scale*. This consists of six sub-tests, viz. information, comprehension, arithmetic, similarities, digit span (a test of immediate recall of numbers forward and backward) and vocabulary.

(b) *Performance Scale*. This consists of five sub-tests, viz. *digit symbol*, in which symbols are linked with numbers and in a given time the subject writes the symbols in blank spaces, each of which has a number as the guide; *picture completion*, in which the subject has to identify the missing part of a picture; *block design*, in which the subject has to arrange coloured blocks in the form of a design which is represented on a card; *picture arrangement*, in which pictures have to be arranged in a sequence to tell a story; *object assembly*, which consists of pieces of cardboard which fit together like a jig-saw to form a face, hand or animal.

A verbal I.Q., performance I.Q. and full-scale I.Q. is finally scored. This test is also useful in the assessment of intellectual deterioration.

There is a form of the test which is suitable for children (WISC).

Which tests are useful for **measuring intellectual deterioration?**

1. *Babcock*

The subject's Stanford-Binet vocabulary score is used to estimate his expected performance on a series of tests of memory, learning and motor speed. The difference between the actual and estimated score is calculated and quantified as an 'Efficiency Index'.

2. *Shipley-Hartford*

Based on the Babcock Scale but simpler to administer and score. It consists of a vocabulary scale and an 'abstraction' scale. The difference between these two scales is finally assessed, after reference to tables as a 'Conceptual Quotient'.

3. *WAIS*

In patients with intellectual deterioration, there tends to be a specific pattern, in that the performance sub-tests show much lower scores than the vocabulary sub-tests. The scatter of scores on the various sub-tests is useful in evaluating particular areas of intellectual deficit.

4. *Tests of abstract conceptual thought*

Several of the performance sub-tests of the WAIS fulfil this function, as also does the Kohs Blocks Test, which is similar in principle to the block design sub-test of the WAIS. Goldstein elaborated a series of tests specifically for the brain damaged subject.

Goldstein-Scheerer Cube—similar to Kohs Blocks.

Gelb-Goldstein Sorting—woollen strands are sorted according to their colour, and matching is also done.

Variations of Goldstein's tests exist and are associated with the names of Vigotsky, Hanfmann and Kasanin.

5. *Perceptual tests*

Bender-Gestalt is based on Gestalt psychology and employs a series of designs and patterns. The subject has to copy designs, and this ability, taking into account the form, shape, irregularity and gap-filling ('closure'), is quantified in a score.

6. *Tests of memory and learning*

There are numerous memory scales, and the processes of learning and memory are tested to some extent in several of the afore-mentioned tests. The *Modified Word Learning Test*, as the name suggests, tests the subject's verbal learning ability. Poor or 'organic' scores are obtained with brain-damaged patients.

Write notes on the commoner psychological **tests of personality**

Personality tests can be divided into two groups; one in which a personality profile is designed in the form of a questionnaire, usually with multiple choice answers, and the other whereby the subject is given an unstructured task, permitting individual responses and flexibility in interpretation.

1. *Questionnaires*

The Minnesota Multiphasic Personality Inventory (MMPI). This comprehensive inventory sets out to evaluate those traits that are commonly characteristic of severe psychiatric disturbance. There are 550 affirmative statements on cards which the patient is asked to place in three stacks—'true', 'false', and 'cannot say'. It may also be used as a group test. A number of scales exist, e.g. for hypochondriasis, depression, hysteria, psychopathy, paranoia, schizophrenia and hypomania.

Maudsley Personality Inventory (MPI) and Eysenck Personality Inventory (EPI). These inventories are very similar and give two measures of personality: *neuroticism* and *extraversion*. Neuroticism is defined by Eysenck as the general emotional lability of the subject, his emotional over-responsiveness and his liability to neurotic breakdown under stress. Extraversion refers to the outgoing social proclivities. Neuroticism scores of 'neurotics' have been found to be consistently and significantly higher than those of normal people.

2. *Projective Tests*

Rorschach. Ink-blots are presented one at a time on 10 cards, five of which are coloured, the other five being in black and grey, and the patient is asked to comment. Scoring is elaborate and probably not helpful in clinical practice where the main use of the test is as a talking point with inhibited patients.

Thematic Apperception Test (TAT). Nineteen cards with black and white pictures and one blank card are presented to the patient, who is asked to construct a story to fit the picture and to interpret the picture. Responses may give a clue to his conflicts, phantasy life, etc.

Both of the above projective tests may be administered as group tests, by making slides of the pictures.

Other projective techniques include word association tests, sentence completion tests, drawing, painting, drama and game-playing with children.

What is a **rating scale** *and give examples of their use in psychiatry?*

The rating scale is a form of clinical measurement for quantifying the signs and symptoms of illness as described by the patient or observed by the doctor. For example, features such as anxiety, depression, hostility, restlessness, delusions and hallucinations can form part of a check-list of clinical features. Each item can be quantified by using a 5-point scale with 0 = absent; 1 = minimal; 2 = moderate; 3 = marked and 4 = severe. Usually instructions accompany a rating scale and each item is defined and the use of the scale explained.

It is a fallacy to consider that a 10-point scale gives a greater degree of accurate measurement than a 5-point scale. It could be the reverse, for the condition which is being measured may not lend itself to such fine observations, and a scale can only be as useful as it is relevant to the problems it measures.

Rating scales are being increasingly used in the clinical evaluation of patients in initial assessment and follow-up as well as in research projects and drug trials, for they allow for comparisons between patient and patient and in the same patient. They are usually classified as:

1. Those completed by a trained observer.

2. Those completed by the patient.

The more common observer scales are:

1. *The Hamilton Rating Scales* for Depression and Anxiety.
   (a) *Depression.* This consists of the following 17 items: depressed mood, guilt, suicidal ideas, initial insomnia, middle insomnia, delayed insomnia, work and interests, retardation, agitation, psychic anxiety, somatic anxiety, gastro-intestinal somatic symptoms, general somatic symptoms, genital symptoms, hypochondriasis, loss of insight and loss of weight. Diurnal variation, depersonalisation, paranoid and obsessional symptoms are mentioned as being worthy of consideration but are not included in the rating score.
   (b) *Anxiety.* This includes 12 features which are commonly found in patients with anxiety states. Each of the following items is rated in degree of severity: anxious mood, tension, fears, insomnia, intellect, depressed mood, general somatic, cardiovascular, respiratory, gastro-intestinal, genito-urinary, autonomic, and behaviour at interview.

2. *Shapiro's Personal Questionnaire.* This is designed to assess psychological *changes* in the same patient and is used for intensive individual studies.

3. *The Lorr Scale.* This has a total of 75 items which cover a large variety of psychiatric symptoms and descriptions of mood and behaviour.

4. *The Wittenborn Scale* contains 72 items or scales and differs from the Lorr on two main points:

(a) Completion of the scales is not restricted to only one interview, thereby allowing more extensive observation and taking into account the variability and episodic nature of some psychiatric symptoms and signs.

(b) Almost every item is rated on a 4-point scale, each grading being associated with a descriptive sentence.

The more commonly used self-rating scales are:

1. *The Minnesota Multiphasic Personality Inventory or MMPI* (*vide supra*).

2. *The Taylor Manifest Anxiety Scale* which measures various anxiety items as in the Hamilton Anxiety Scale, but it is assessed by the patient himself.

3. *Beck's Depression Inventory* and 4. *Zung's Depression Scale.*

These contain items similar to the Hamilton Scale for Depression but are self-rating. Other examples include questionnaires on hostility and direction of hostility. For self-rating scales to be employed, the patient must be sufficiently co-operative and well enough to complete a self-reporting form.

A more recent development is the use of a self-rating scale for depression (or anxiety) involving a visual analogue scale. In this, the patient marks a line of arbitrary length according to the degree of his emotional feelings.

Rating scales in psychiatry can be criticised on the grounds that the phenomenology and natural history of disease in psychiatry has not yet been firmly established and agreed. In some instances they are merely an attempt to quantify adjectives with nouns missing.

What is meant by Grid Techniques?

Grid Techniques or repertory grids have evolved from Kelly's work on 'personal constructs' as represented in his book *The Psychology of Personal Constructs*. His basic assumption is that to understand an individual's psychological make-up it is necessary to find out how he views or construes the world around him. One can for instance investigate in which way the individual distinguishes between people close to him, and how he regards them as sharing certain characteristics. By extending the individual's considerations to various people, objects, situations and human characteristics, a more complete picture can be gained of his 'constructs'. Thus, in any individual case, an arbitrary series of constructs can be completed. Kelly proposed that if any of a person's most important constructs were stressed or disrupted in any way, then conditions were ripe for the development of mental disorder.

Grid techniques involve the application and recording of the individual's constructs in the interview situation. The interview is thus a structured one. Various 'elements' are selected, e.g. people, events, and choice of objects in everyday life. These elements are then compared by the individual being tested, who evaluates them by using 'constructs'. The results are recorded numerically in a table with a row for every construct and a column for every element. The term 'grid' applies to the completed table. Grid techniques have been further developed to examine such diverse phenomena as changes in attitude following psychotherapy and thought disorder in schizophrenic patients. The numerical nature of grids allows statistical manipulation of results and computer handling.

A related method is the *semantic differential*. This also investigates the nature of a person's concepts, but while grid technique is suitable for individual cases, the semantic differential is more applicable to groups or samples of people. Although some purists in the sphere of psychology maintain that grids and the semantic differential are poles apart on theoretical grounds at least, the general consensus of opinion is that a semantic differential is a grid described in different terms. Neither method has as yet become clinically established.

SECTION 2

PSYCHOPATHOLOGY

What is meant by **psychopathology?**

Though it means mental pathology or pathology of the mind, it is now defined as study of the mental processes which underlie mental illness.

History

Though others had made earlier contributions, it was *Sigmund Freud*, the Viennese doctor, at the end of the nineteenth century, who gave the most comprehensive account of these processes. He based his theories on the principle that the mind had an *Unconscious* as well as a *Conscious* component, i.e. there is a large part of mental life or function of which we are not consciously aware. Evidence of this is found in:

(a) slips of the tongue, selective forgetting and other aspects of everyday life;

(b) hysterical symptoms which are considered to be due to a form of mental dissociation, i.e. a splitting off a part from the main stream of consciousness;

(c) the phenomenon of hypnosis where part of mental functioning can be split off from the main stream, as in hysteria;

(d) dream analysis. The manifest content of the dream is all the sleeper is able to recall but during analysis much of the latent content can be uncovered, indicating that unconscious aspects of mental life were operating in the dream experience.

What are the constituents of the **unconscious?**

1. The *id* which is derived from the German neutral pronoun '*das Es*' or 'It'. Freud regarded this as the source of the infant's instinctive drives for food, sex and aggressive impulses which demand immediate satisfaction. It is amoral and egocentric; ruled by the pleasure-pain principle in that it does what it likes and avoids what it finds unpleasant; is without a sense of time; is

22

completely illogical; primarily sexual; infantile in its emotional status; will not take 'no' for an answer; is without verbal representation and therefore does not enter consciousness. The portrayal of the new-born child as the prime example of the id-ridden individual is underlined by the following amusing definition of the new-born child: 'an alimentary tract with no sense of responsibility at either end'.

This lack of responsibility is not allowed to persist and society through parents, teachers and others begins to impose its morality and code of behaviour on the child.

2. This aspect of the unconscious is called the *super-ego*. Though inaccessible to the ego it exercises some control over it. Though a neighbour of the id in the individual's unconscious, it is frequently disapproving and is the moral critic which is responsible for the sense of guilt borne by the ego. It is more rigid than the traditional voice of conscience. A super-ego which is developed in a background of fear and punishment is claimed to make for a more brittle ego than one which is based on identification and introjection of the standards of parents and teachers.

What is the 'Oedipus complex'?

This is a term derived from Greek mythology to explain the conflict arising from an unconscious desire for the individual to possess the parent of the opposite sex. This impulse which is common to all in their psychosexual development is repressed at an early stage and becomes incorporated in the super-ego. In some societies it is contained entirely in a strong social taboo with its many ramifications. In our society it rests with the super-ego and conflict can be reactivated by external events.

What is the ego?

Though largely conscious it has strong links with the unconscious. It uses logic; deals with the outer world; is usually influenced by the super-ego; has moral standards; has time perception; is verbalised; and sleeps but has a dream censorship. It makes contact with the environment through the sensory processes and is able to evaluate the information and effect compromises. It therefore has to modify the impulses of the id

B

and is or should be concerned with the *reality principle*. It therefore represents the personality of the individual to the observer.

What are **ego-defences?**

To understand what is meant by ego-defences it is necessary to appreciate that the ego may be strong or weak. Ego-strength is said to arise from secure early relationships which permit the personality to develop without the brittleness or defects which a less secure background may produce. Such a background ensures an adequate quota of resistance to external stresses as well as a lessening of the individual's need to expose himself to them. This latter point requires stating for it is not sufficiently appreciated that there are a number of people who are invariably unlucky, are always getting hurt and are never successful. Though external factors may appear to explain their misfortunes, there is a strong inner compulsion which repeatedly exposes them to hazards. This tendency is said to be due to early influences on the ego which have predisposed it to this form of behaviour. It could be regarded as a form of ego-weakness.

It is when the ego is having difficulty in coping with internal or external problems that certain defence mechanisms are employed. A strong ego need not resort to such defences and will react to stress in a normal healthy manner without displaying any mental abnormality. Should there be evidence of such abnormality it *may* mean that the ego is not coping adequately, but this is not necessarily so, for an ego-defence mechanism which is very much in evidence may provide adequate compensation for the stress and the individual is not in the least handicapped. In such cases, the ego is said to be *well-compensated*; if the defence is inadequate, the ego is said to be *decompensating*.

Describe the commoner **ego-defence mechanisms**

1. *Dissociation.* This is said to occur when the ego divorces itself from the conflict by converting the anxiety into physical or mental incapacity. This 'flight into functional incapacity' which is usually referred to as *hysteria* used to be a very common condition and could be regarded as a distress signal which not only relieved the individual of his anxiety but would also draw the attention of society to his problem.

Dissociation or hysterical behaviour is still common in other cultures and it can present in a variety of ways such as loss of use of limbs, blindness, loss of memory and regressed or infantile behaviour.

2. *Projection.* This is a tendency, sometimes masked, to externalise personal insecurities and the person frequently blames others for his own shortcomings. This attitude may be a basic personality trait, in that some people are always accusing others of hostile intent, and is not inconsistent with adequate ego-strength. There are many very able and successful people of this stamp, who by their drive and ability make useful contributions to society. It is when the mechanism appears for the first time and catches the observer by surprise, or becomes markedly aggravated with frankly delusional talk that decompensation should be suspected.

Even when faced with the most fantastic stories one should not jump to the conclusion that the person is using the mechanism of projection. Every statement should be carefully and objectively assessed for some very strange and unlikely stories have been proved true.

3. *Obsessional features.* These may constitute a personality trait which is frequently within the range of normal behaviour and can be highly desirable. It may consist of such a scrupulous attitude to tidiness, punctuality and duty that the individual who exhibits the trait becomes a most invaluable person in any organisation. Even when the mechanism goes well beyond what might be considered the normal range, it may be compatible, not only with efficiency, but with professional eminence. Ritual hand-washing, 'obsessional' note-taking, and 'obsessional' politeness can all be borne by some individuals without any evidence of ego-disintegration or loss of efficiency. The mechanism itself, as with projection, can become an ego-strengthener, and many successful people show it to a marked degree.

The mechanism can however be invoked to bolster up a disintegrating ego, particularly in the young, and any recent exaggeration of the trait with consequent loss of efficiency is likely to indicate the beginnings of decompensation.

4. *Ego-mutilation.* It may seem paradoxical to include a process which mutilates the ego under 'ego-defences'. This mechanism is invoked when the ego is under severe stress and something has

got to give. Instead of a complete ego-disintegration there is a sacrifice of part of the person's ego which may be represented by eccentric behaviour or affectation in speech, dress or some mannerism. The individual, while retaining the essential ingredients of his personality and his contact with reality, nevertheless behaves or looks queer. It is no accident of speech that some patterns of behaviour associated with the sexual perversion of homosexuality are also referred to as 'queer' for they are essentially eccentricities based on ego-mutilation.

5. *Denial.* This is frequently invoked where the individual has to live with a distressing or painful problem with which he is unable to cope. He denies its existence and behaves as if it is not there or is not nearly as grave as he is told. It is seen commonly in the parents of schizophrenics who may claim that all is well and deny that their child is mentally ill. It is likely that the only way they can live with the problem is to deny it. A similar mechanism may be used by those who live intimately for many years with deluded patients.

6. *Undoing.* This is seen in everyday life in such common practices as handshaking which is designed to control aggression. It is the basis of ritualistic or superstitious acts in both adults and children and consists of something positive being done which actually or magically is the opposite of the forbidden impulse and thus cancels it. Its place in obsessional features is obvious.

7. *Isolation.* This mechanism is designed to keep thought and feeling apart. It is essential for logical thinking, for, by excluding the charged feeling aspect, logical thought can proceed. Most objects in addition to their actual meaning have a symbolic meaning which is emotionally charged. The latter may obtrude during sleep but in consciousness the symbolism is isolated.

8. *Reaction formation.* Instead of repeated attempts at repression to deal with dangerous impulses arising from the unconscious, the ego reacts against them by presenting the opposite side. Excessive cleanliness and tidiness may be a defence against the impulse to soil; excessive kindness against cruelty; excessive generosity against acquisitiveness. These in addition to containing the undesirable impulse help the child to become socially acceptable, and, like isolation and undoing, play a part in character formation.

9. *Repression.* The impulses arising from the id are not always permitted to reach consciousness, and, if too disturbing, are repressed and return to the unconscious. Most of what is repressed in early life remains repressed, but in adolescence many of the infantile taboos are lifted and some of these impulses again seek expression in consciousness and may give rise to conflict.

10. *Identification.* This is a very important mechanism in the development of the child. It permits the incorporation of the qualities of parents and parent substitutes and thus contributes to character formation. In the adult it occurs as a defence mechanism in times of stress such as bereavement or fantasied loss and he may then turn to a person or cult and become slavishly identified.

11. *Displacement.* The repressed impulse may be displaced to another object or situation. This second choice is more acceptable to the ego than the first which has been repudiated. In children the mechanism is entirely unconscious but in adults there is an element of choice.

12. *Rationalisation.* People tend to explain their behaviour in a manner which is acceptable to their 'ego ideal' rather than give the 'naked truth' which may well reveal their selfish and un-principled motives and thus make themeselves appear objectionable in their own estimation and in that of society. It is a very common mechanism which is readily resorted to by people in public life and is found in situations where primitive impulses are released, such as in domestic quarrels. Some would deride all altruism as rationalisation; this is not so, and merely indicates the abuse of a superficial knowledge of mental mechanisms.

What is meant by **ego-disintegration**?

If the ego is unable to hold the line even with the exploitation of its defence mechanisms, ego-disintegration may occur. As dissociation, projection, undoing and eccentricity may have already been exploited, though in vain, their broken-down ramparts may be apparent in addition to the change in personality which is the essential feature of ego-disintegration. Concomitant with the breakdown in the defence is a regression to a more infantile pattern of behaviour, speech and thought and a greater divorcement from reality. This leads to the protean manifestation of a condition which has been given the name *schizophrenia*.

Discuss the libido theory of neurosis

This theory is based on Freud's concept that the libido is the source of energy which is attached to the sexual instinct. Originally Freud regarded the sex instinct as it is understood in the everyday sense, but he later applied it to any pleasurable sensation relating to the bodily function and also through the process of *sublimation*, to socially approved forms of behaviour such as fellow-feeling and enjoyment of work and social responsibilities. Adult sex drives need not therefore be directed towards persons of the opposite sex and neither, for that matter, is genital union necessarily the object of sexual behaviour. He pointed out the chronological sequence that such attachments follow and defined three phases:

1. *The oral phase*

This starts at birth and continues for approximately 18 months, and oral eroticism is said to stem from the pleasure the infant derives from breast feeding. When the breast is withdrawn, alternative sources of erotic 'nourishment' are sought and in infancy these include thumb-sucking or putting other objects into the mouth. This oral eroticism persists into adult life in the form of kissing, smoking and eating as well as in overt sexual perversions. Although in infancy the libido is primarily fixated at an oral level, it is, in earliest infancy, diffusely spread all over the body and auto-eroticism is paramount; this narcissism may persist into adult life. In early infancy the ego is undifferentiated, i.e. it has not yet reached the stage when it can distinguish 'self' from 'not self' and the first love-object, the breast, may be regarded by the infant as an extension of itself. It is only when it is withdrawn that this universality of self is broken and external love-objects are identified. The early oral phase is a passive one, but when the child acquires teeth it assumes a more aggressive role.

2. *The anal phase*

This overlaps the oral one and is said to continue till three years. Erotogenic zones are anus, rectum and bladder, and pleasure is derived from excretion and later retention of urine and faeces. It is then that an ambivalent attitude develops towards adults who both thwart and gratify the child's desires, and characteristics such as cleanliness, neatness and punctuality are also established.

3. *The phallic phase*

This overlaps the anal one and continues to develop till the child is about 7 years old. There are naturally differences between the sexes.

(a) *In boys*, awareness of penis sensitivity may lead to masturbation at an early age and associated fantasies are usually of the mother. The father is seen as a rival for the mother's love and the boy develops hostile thoughts towards him. This is referred to as the *Oedipus complex* after the main character in Sophocles' tragedy, *Oedipus Rex* who killed his father and married his mother without knowing the identity of either. The working through of the Oedipus situation is a very important part of psychosexual development which is usually completed by the fourth to fifth year. At about the same time the boy becomes aware of the female lack of a penis which in association with his guilt over the Oedipus situation creates a fear of punishment which is referred to as '*castration anxiety*'.

(b) *In girls*, the situation is more complex. The discovery of a penis in the male creates what is called '*penis envy*' and this is associated with a tendency to blame the mother for depriving her of this object. It is then that she turns from her mother to her father and has fantasies of getting from him either a penis or a baby and the mother becomes her rival for the father's love. This has been called the *Electra complex* again from a Greek myth in which Electra connives at the death of her mother Clytemnestra who had murdered her father Agamemnon. It is said to occur when the girl has renounced the hope of masculinity and reconciled herself to castration as an accepted fact.

The working through of the Oedipus situation marks the end of infantile sexuality, while an unconscious tendency to perpetuate Oedipal strivings forms the basis for many neurotic processes.

4. *The latency period*

This occurs between 7 and 12 years or the onset of puberty. During it the Oedipus situation is resolved and a stronger super-ego is developed, with increased moral responsibility. Curiosity is directed into non-sexual channels and the child makes rapid progress in scholastic and physical activities. It is during this period that group loyalties such as group membership and hero worship outside the family circle (usually for someone of the same sex) occur.

In adolescence the sex instinct is strongly re-awakened, with consequent masturbation and interest in the opposite or same sex, depending on the degree of resolution of the Oedipal situation. Much of this increased sexual activity is of course due to hormonal changes.

Libido-direction

This not only varies in its localisation such as anal, oral and genital, but also in its object choice and here too it goes through stages. The first is *auto-erotic*, where the child is both lover and loved one and this is entirely an *id* activity. The second is *narcissistic* which occurs when the ego is differentiated from external reality; self-awareness results and libidinal impulses are self-directed. This process may persist into adult life. These two stages, both meaning self-love are not identical. The former is independent of the concept of a personality and is really a form of animal self-stimulation. Narcissism, though mediating through auto-eroticism, is a sequel of ego-differentiation. A third stage is *allo-eroticism*, which is the seeking of a love-object outside oneself and is at the core of the Oedipus situation.

The fate of the libido

It can be *allo-erotic* or *narcissistic* and the latter can be *primary* as already described, or *secondary*, where the libido is frustrated and turned in on the ego which is now identified as a love-object. This can be a normal experience but it can also be evidence of severe mental disorder. The libido can also be *fixated*. Normally there is a progression of love-objects from mother to mate, but arrest can occur at any time at the mother or mother-substitute level. It can also *regress*, which implies previous maturity, but in the face of a traumatic situation the libido has returned to an earlier love-object from which it had derived greater security. It may be *repressed* which is a defensive mechanism to prevent the flooding of consciousness with painful or distasteful material. Repression is used to keep the normal quota of homosexuality under control, so that the average person who is neither a latent nor overt homosexual can be said to be an effectively repressed one. Lastly the libido may be *sublimated* or expressed in a socially approved form where the energy of the sex desire is directed into non-sexual channels. Great social contributions such as the creative activity of artists have been attributed to sublimation.

Summarise **Freud's theory of dreams**

Freud regarded dreams as the mode of reaction of the mind to stimuli acting on it during sleep, though these stimuli need not be exclusively psychological. He laid down the following three basic principles in dream interpretation:

1. The function of the dream is to preserve sleep.
2. There is a latent as well as a manifest content and it is frequently the former which is the more significant.
3. The dream represents the gratification of an unfulfilled wish which is usually infantile.

Dream analysis therefore gives clues to repressed urges which were disguised by the manifest content. In the waking state censorship or repression is more effective, but in sleep it is alleged to be relaxed and an impasse in therapy can often be resolved by dream analysis.

Efforts to disguise the dream's latent content are called *the dream work* and Freud described four mechanisms whereby it operates. The first three are regressive with archaic forms of expression showing conspicuous absence of abstract thinking. They are:

1. *Dramatisation,* where abstract ideas are given solid or concrete shape with the free use of symbols representing repressed activities or experiences.
2. *Condensation,* which is a form of abbreviation or shorthand which conceals from the dreamer some of the latent content by omission, or by using a part, sometimes a very small part, to

represent a whole, or by the fusing of a variety of latent elements sharing a common feature into one piece.

3. *Displacement*, which is the replacement of the latent content by a remotely associated element which is no more than an allusion or oblique reference, or shifting the accent so that the latent content is barely recognisable.

4. *Secondary elaboration*, which occurs just as full consciousness is regained and continues for a time during the waking state, thus making the dream appear more rational.

Dream interpretation

This is practised by using free-association to convert the manifest content to latent, and the material produced is handled as neurotic symptoms, on the assumption that each dream represents a wish, probably infantile, which the patient cannot tolerate in the waking state, but in its disguised form can achieve gratification and sleep.

Dream symbols

These are used by the dreamers as a form of camouflage. A selected sample are: exalted persons such as kings and queens (or the modern equivalent) for parents; references to water for birth; going on a journey for dying; clothes or uniform for nakedness or shame; the number three for male genitalia; long, straight objects like poles, trees, sticks or sharp objects like daggers, or guns and revolvers for the phallus.

Discuss briefly the contributions to medical psychology of C. G. Jung and Alfred Adler

Analytical psychology (C. G. Jung)

This was founded by C. G. Jung (1875-1961), who was an early associate of Freud but after a few years broke with the psycho-analytic movement as he had ascribed to the unconscious functions which were considered beyond those necessary for orthodox psychoanalytic theory. He was keenly interested in symbols and found during analysis that some recurred more frequently than others and were common to a variety of cultures, particularly in myths and legends. Jung considered that these were not part of the individual's personal experience but were, like his body, made up of his racial past and profoundly influenced behaviour, forming part of the *racial* or *collective unconscious* as opposed to the personal one. This accent on race has been misconstrued by those obsessed with racial theory and particularly supremacy, but it is unlikely that Jung subscribed to this view and he would appear rather to be pleading for the appreciation of a number of 'experiences' in our unconscious which could not have got there post-natally. These he called *archetypes* which, though showing some cultural differences, had universal application. Examples are gods, witches, demons and spirits which are punitive and devouring; the eternal compassionate mother; and magic numbers or geometrical designs such as the mandala, a four-sided figure with a central circle. Personality he regarded as the *persona* or mask worn by Roman actors and was therefore that part of consciousness exposed to the gaze of the world. Those aspects of mental life which are denied in consciousness develop in the unconscious and form the personal unconscious or 'shadow', which plays an important part in dreams and is explained in terms of Jungian typology.

Psychological types

These, which form one of Jung's major studies, were based on two attitudes, extraversion and introversion, and originally to each he ascribed a fundamental function, to the former, feeling and to the latter, thought. This does not mean that the introvert is incapable of feeling or the extravert of thought, but that these functions are unconscious. When the introvert is faced with a situation demanding feeling rather than thought, a conflict arises because of tension between these opposing faculties. Jung later modified this relatively simple plan by ascribing the four functions, thinking, feeling, intuition and sensation, to each individual, and qualifying them as 'superior' and 'inferior', with thought and feeling, intuition and sensation as paired opposites. Diagrammatically, if thought were 'superior', feeling was 'inferior', with sensation and intuition coming in between. The scheme was further complicated by introducing empirical thinking between thinking and sensation, emotional feeling between sensation and feeling, intuitive feeling between feeling and intuition, and speculative thinking between intuition and thinking. Add to these the attitudes extraversion and introversion, and the mariner's compass loses on points!

Jung laid great stress on dream analysis, but his interpretations, while in some respects similar to those of Freud, took into account the archetypes and he dismissed the idea of a censorship preventing the emergence of unconscious material into consciousness. He regarded a symbol as not only evidence of repression but an attempt to point out the way to the dreamer. The Jungian analyst is expected to use his knowledge of anthropology and world classical literature to interpret dreams and is not restricted by the dreamer's personal inexperience of these data, for, he argues, they are part of his collective or racial unconscious. Analysis of the personal unconscious is therefore only the first part of the treatment; the second and more difficult is that of the racial unconscious. The libido is seen differently too, as a primal and universal force corresponding to Bergson's *élan vital*.

The psyche is said to have an unconscious presentation which is the sexual counterpart of the true sexual expression of the individual and either sex may project its opposite. The feminine unconscious persona is called the *anima* and the male the *animus*. Because Jung considered the woman to be monogamous, her animus is multiform and George Eliot, the authoress, is quoted as an example of an active and multiform animus which is projected into her writings.

Criticisms

Jung's methodology has been criticised because of its logical inconsistencies. It argues that because *A* is somewhat like *B* and *B* can, under certain circumstances, share something with *C*, and *C* has been known on occasions to have been suspected to being related to *D*, the conclusion in full-fledged logical form is that *A=D*. As the language of science this is meaningless.

One gets the same impression from reading Jung as might be obtained from reading the scriptures of the Hindus, Taoists or Confucius; although well aware that many wise and true things are being said, one feels that they could have been said just as well without involving one in the psychological theories upon which they are supposedly based.

Although Jung has not had anything like the impact on medical psychology as Freud, he has a fascination for theologians and a number have adopted Jung's theories in their 'pastoral psychology' or more generally in their mission of healing.

Individual psychology of Adler

This is the name given to the system of psychology devised by Alfred Adler (1870-1937). He was the first of Freud's associates to break away and establish his own theory which he regarded as a key to the understanding of the whole of mental life. He expressed his basic tenet thus: 'To be a human being means the possession of a feeling of inferiority that is constantly pressing on towards its own conquest'. His writings are strongly influenced by Nietzschean philosophy, and terms such as 'organ inferiority' with strivings to over-compensate for this inferiority, and the 'will to power' are frequently referred to. He considered that man has to make major adjustments to society, vocation and love, and his capacity to make these would depend on childhood experiences and the 'life-style' patterned on them. He explained that the helplessness of the child gives it an 'inferiority complex' which can be accentuated by an organ inferiority or unsuitable early handling such as spoiling, sarcasm or snubbing. Inferiority is dealt with by the individual in three ways: (1) by successful compensation, as, for example, Beethoven with his deafness and Demosthenes with his stammer; (2) defeat is followed by retreat, which is regarded as the normal pattern in some cultures; (3) compromise or over-compensation, the former being a tendency to attribute the failure to the physical inferiority, while the latter is a ridiculous protest against it. Examples of the latter are the little man who is always aggressive and challenging, and the dull man who affects an intellectual pose. Over-compensation can result in decompensation and neurosis.

Adler used the term 'neurosis' in an all-embracing sense and paid no heed to differences in diagnosis. He made sweeping generalisations, such as 'every neurosis can be understood as an attempt to free oneself from a feeling of inferiority in order to gain a feeling of superiority'. His concept of aetiology was not localised in the unconscious but in the child's environment and family style. The inferior organ he regarded as occasionally conditioned by psychological factors and serving as a defence mechanism, and in practically all illness he defined three factors: the structural, the functional and the psychic, the last being the major one in neurotic illness. This concept has found a place in the field of psycho-somatic medicine, but as with many speculations, adequate proof is elusive. The idea of 'organ jargon', where the inferior or affected part is in fact communicating its psychological stress, is an Adlerian concept. Neurotic or delinquent behaviour may stem from the child's erroneous solution to its problems. Over-compensation may result in a phantasy goal which is virtually unattainable and give rise to abnormal behaviour patterns, or to much compensatory day-dreaming and withdrawal from reality.

Treatment is largely a matter of imparting insight and depends on a painstaking analysis of the early childhood experiences and life and family 'styles', paying particular attention to birth rank, sibling rivalry, family careers and adverse environmental factors. An appreciation of the patient's strivings or *'masculine protest'* would then emerge and repetition of behaviour patterns become evident. Efforts to overcome the handicap include advice and even practical help, for the Adlerian does not adhere to the detached 'scientific' attitude of the psychoanalyst. It is not surprising therefore, that social rehabilitation units, out-patient social clubs and day hospitals have been largely inspired by Adlerian theory, though it could be argued that such expedients would have evolved in any case. It is essentially a system of psychology for the teacher and the 'practical' doctor who have a high regard for the role of environment in the production and removal of neurotic illness. Like other analytical therapies, it requires knowledge and experience, though, as it does not involve 'depth' processes, personal analysis is not essential.

Although Adler has formally had nothing like the influence on psychotherapy as Freud, much of his teaching has been incorporated by others and even Freudian analysts now pay more attention to the ego and non-sexual factors in the causation of neurosis. His methods appeal to those searching for shorter techniques in psychotherapy.

Discuss the major **post-Freudian schools** *of psychotherapy*

H. S. Sullivan (1892-1949). He was an American-born psychiatrist who had a unique understanding of schizophrenia and made important contributions to its psychotherapy. He itemised personality development in the following way:

1. *Infancy*. Empathy is the important influence; an increasing awareness of self; realisation of one's capacities.

2. *Childhood*. Follows infancy and is distinguished by the acquiring of language; cultural indoctrination begins and thought processes are evident; clashes occur between the parent and child.

3. *Juvenile*. Co-operation with compeers; group solidarity; competition and the desire to belong.

4. *Pre-adolescence*. From 8½ years to 12 years (or early puberty). Egocentricity gives way to social responsibility and personal friends are regarded as important as oneself.

5. *Adolescence*. Subdivided into (*a*) early, (*b*) mid (onset of genital behaviour), (*c*) late (establishment of durable intimate relationships).

6. *Maturity*.

Empathy. This term is used by Sullivan to describe the 'emotional contagion or communion' which the child has for its mother or nurse and is particularly evident between the sixth and twenty-seventh months. It may give rise to feeding difficulties which are engendered by the mother's emotional distress and is said to occur also in animals and to be independent of the ordinary sensory channels. Empathy, by making the child aware of its mother's emotional states, is subjected to her reaction to the child's failure to control micturition and defaecation and this may play an important part in habit training. Similarly her approval for good performance will be reflected in the communicative release of her tension.

The self

Once this has developed, it tends to maintain its own form and direction as a system whose basic function is to avoid anxiety. Earliest experiences are most deep-seated and pervasive and though at a later stage the individual may question and compare his experiences he never escapes those early influences. This 'homeostasis' of the 'self' is due to the production of anxiety by experiences which threaten to disrupt or come into conflict with its organisation and the institution of behaviour designed to nullify this anxiety. In Freudian terms this is equivalent to a mobilisation of the ego-defences, but Sullivan used the analogy of the amoeba which digests meat and rejects glass, even when the glass is coated with meat extract. The self-structure is built up during the formative years and thereafter is determined to maintain its integrity, even should it be a poor one.

The self-system

This is the part of the personality which can be observed. True-self is the core of potential which may or may not have been developed and is influenced by cultural factors, since man is moulded by his culture and attempts to break with it produce anxiety. Modifications in later life are possible by people with whom the individual identifies such as parents, teachers and friends and as the self is the sum of 'reflected appraisals', what we think of ourselves may depend on what others have thought of us.

Parataxic distortion

This is the mechanism whereby one may attribute to others traits taken from significant people in one's past. This goes on in most inter-personal relationships so that what is overt does not incorporate all that really goes on between them. The interpretation and removal of these distortions is one of the main purposes of Sullivan's psychotherapy. The patient's evaluations may be compared with those of the psychotherapist on the principle that if one's views differ from those of a person one esteems, these views may be changed. These changes are unlikely to occur in frankly delusional situations but can be effected where neurotic interpretations exist and when insight is possible such as in parataxic distortion.

Karen Horney (1885-1952). She pointed out that many of Freud's basic assumptions were determined by the prevailing philosophical beliefs of his century:

    (*a*) biological orientation;
    (*b*) ignorance of modern anthropology and sociology;
    (*c*) tendency to dualistic thinking;
    (*d*) deliberate abstention from moral judgments;
    (*e*) mechanistic-evolutionistic thinking;

and that deep analytical interpretations which are connected only with infantile drives is a dangerous illusion for the following reasons:

1. It gives a false impression of human relationships, the nature of neurotic conflicts and the role of cultural factors.

2. It pretends that a machine can be understood out of one wheel instead of by a study of the interrelation of all parts.

3. It leads the therapist to assume final limitations to therapy (based on biological factors) when they do not exist.

She also rejects the concept of a universal normal psychology, for behaviour which is regarded as neurotic in one culture may be regarded as normal elsewhere, but she accepts two traits which are present in all neurotics.

1. *Rigidity in reaction.* While normal people have a flexibility suited to their environment, the neurotic tends to react in predetermined ways, e.g. suspicion in the normal is engendered by the environment, while the neurotic brings his suspiciousness with him.

2. *Discrepancy between potentialities and accomplishments.* The individual may be frustrated by harsh realities which cause him to fail in spite of himself, but the neurotic brings about his own failure.

She described the neurosis as: 'a psychic disturbance brought about by fears and defences against these fears, and by attempts to find compromise solutions for conflicting tendencies'.

She also described neurosis as a basic anxiety where one feels small, insignificant, helpless and endangered in a world that is out to abuse, cheat, attack, humiliate, betray and envy. Such feelings are present in children whose parents are incapable of genuine warmth and affection and have therefore never experienced 'the blissful certainty of being wanted'.

In the child's efforts to escape from this anxiety, the following neurotic personality trends are developed:

1. Neurotic striving for affection.
2. Neurotic striving for power.
3. Neurotic withdrawal.
4. Neurotic submissiveness.

Erich Fromm (1900-   ).   He is a sociologist as well as an analyst who was profoundly influenced by Karl Marx and analysed Freudian theory in Marxist terms.   He gave historical examples of how man and his nature varied as between the Middle Ages and the Renaissance, but did not accept that man is entirely moulded by his environment and challenged those like Marx who would 'reduce the psychological facts to a shadow of culture patterns'.

Evolution in man has produced entirely new qualities which have separated him even more from other animals.   He has this awareness of being a separate being, can store the knowledge of the past, visualise the future and through his imagination he reaches far beyond the range of his senses.   Fromm regarded him as a freak of nature.

He traced the history of man from his emergence from a state of oneness with nature which has protected him from loneliness, though he is blocked as a free self-determining productive individual.   By the Middle Ages he had lost his feelings of unity with nature though he still had social solidarity.   The free market did not operate and personal, economic and social life was governed by rules laid down by the Church.   With the Renaissance individualism emerged in all classes and pervaded all forms of activity and with this new-found freedom, emotional security was lost.   This was accentuated with the growth of Protestantism which became closely identified with the new Capitalism.   Man constantly longs for the Golden Age when he was at one with the world and did not have to bear the heavy burden of individual freedom.   Modern totalitarianism has tried to woo man from his freedom by offering him membership of a uniform (literally) group.   Industrial society with its mergers and other arrangements makes it more and more difficult for the individual to impose any rational order on things or even to identify with a group.   The individual elaborates the following psychic mechanisms to overcome his problems:

1. Moral masochism.
2. Sadism.
3. Destructiveness.
4. Automaton conformity.

5. Love. This he regards as a normal approach, the previous four being neurotic.

He also elaborated the following character traits:

1. The receptive.
2. The exploitative.
3. The hoarding.
4. The marketing.
5. The productive.

While Marxist theory may no longer be applicable to the economic problems of our time, Fromm has introduced a freshness of outlook into psychopathology which not only takes into account cultural factors, but provides a contemporary analogy which is recognisable. It is not particularly helpful in the understanding of the severer forms of mental illness, but is useful in providing a framework for character types and assessing the 'life-style'.

Otto Rank (1884-1939). He was impressed by the similarities of the physiological concomitants of anxiety and those accompanying birth, and because of this denied that the Oedipus complex occupied the central position in the aetiology of neurosis but considered that all neurosis originated in the birth trauma, which in essence is separation from the mother. Further separation experiences such as weaning (separation from the breast) and symbolic castration (separation from the penis) or separation from a loved object or person could reactivate this anxiety. He divided this anxiety into two forms:

1. *The life fear*. This occurs when the individual becomes aware of creative capacities within himself which if asserted would threaten him with independence and therefore the separation from existing relationships.

2. *The death fear*. This is the fear of losing one's individuality and being swallowed up in the whole.

Throughout life each person is spurred foward by the need to express his individuality yet is restrained by the fear that by doing so he may cut himself off from society. Two solutions are possible:

1. *Normal*, or the wholehearted acceptance of society's standards as one's own.

2. *Creative*, or standing alone and producing one's own standards.

The neurotic can accept neither.

Like Fromm, he saw society as both patriarchal and matriarchal, and religion in terms of sublimation of the fears of the primal birth trauma.   Resurrection is therefore a conquering of the birth trauma and Paradise is a return to the mother and her protecting womb.

What is **existential psychiatry?**

This derives from the Existentialist movement in philosophy which in its modern setting starts with Kierkegaard's reaction against the rationalism of Hegel and his insistence that truth could be found only in existence. He agitated against the theology and practice of the state church on the grounds that religion was for the individual soul and should be separated from the state and the world. A number of psychiatrists, including Binswanger, protested against 'the subject-object cleavage of the world', and in their own reaction against the rationalism and objectivity of the psychoanalytic movement mirrored the reaction of Kierkegaard.

A major contributor to the psychopathological interpretations of existentialism is Sartre who, as an atheist, denied the existence of God and asserted that only Man exists and that his past which includes historical and physical information common to all men is 'non-authentic' and therefore all accent should be placed on the present.

Schizophrenics have received special attention from existentialists. Their main problem is a failure to belong because their weak and tender selves are not suitable for the human society of the natural, strong, domineering and amoral man. The anxiety they carry, their single-mindedness concerning the nature or constitution of the world, their insight, their lack of self-deception and their sense of responsibility are all reminiscent of existentialism. The existential psychiatrist does not regard such a 'pathological' outlook on life as psychotic and may prefer to indict the society which has engendered such a reaction. The patient therefore may not be regarded as sick as the society in which he lives. All this is in accord with *avant-garde* thinking but whether it makes a material contribution to therapy is doubtful though it does make a contribution to the understanding of schizophrenia. It is on this philosophy that R. D. Laing in his books, *The Divided Self* and *The Politics of the Family and other Essays*, has gained his reputation.

Discuss briefly the contribution of **Karl Jaspers**

He sees psychopathology as being chiefly concerned with conscious psychic events though he appreciates that extraconscious mechanisms and unconscious mental processes also play a part. He therefore limits it to the study of the psychic state as experienced by patients and the 'meaningful connexions' within the psyche and the 'causal connexions' between psychic and extrapsychic events. These causal factors he regards as always extrapsychic while abnormal mental phenomena are based on personality development or on an intercurrent illness.

He argues his case with considerable logic and it is understandable that Jaspers has a greater reputation among European (including British) schools of philosophy than with British psychiatrists. It is all oversimplified and though the phenomenology of psychiatric illness is described with great accuracy and detail, Jaspers fails to see that much of it is dependent on the institutional milieu in which the patients then lived. He therefore is unaware of some of the meaningful links, and 'real causes' like genetics, which were considered proven at the time his first edition appeared, are no longer tenable. This work has however greatly influenced German psychiatric thinking, and some who are unhappy over the logical inconsistencies of Freudian psychopathology or who would wish to subscribe to anything but Freud will find in Jaspers an adequate intellectual exercise. It will not help towards an understanding of the apparent illogicalities and contradictions of emotionally toned behaviour and is therefore very dated and out of touch with modern advances in psychiatry.

What is meant by the **myth of mental illness?**

This is the title of a book by Thomas Szasz who takes as his starting point the phenomena grouped under Hysteria. He shows that these and other aspects of mental illness are mainly a form of communication which has in society achieved a degree of understanding and that many non-medical problems are dressed in psychiatric language or jargon because society, including doctors, has decreed that this is acceptable. It thus has many of the qualities of a fashion in that it can assume epidemic proportions and then almost disappear or change its character.

The argument is valid in many examples of hysterical or manipulative behaviour and in the over-emphasis of illness in many common forms of delinquent behaviour, but it is difficult to accept that it has much place in the explanation of psychotic illness, although even here what one may regard as 'psychotic' in one culture may be a manipulative hysterical display in another. As long as psychiatric diagnosis is limited to phenomenology, the 'language of psychiatry' will be used for secondary gain. There is always the danger that should society react against this 'mythology', genuinely sick people will be misunderstood.

Discuss the **validity of psychopathology** in the interpretation of mental phenomena

A scientific evaluation of psychopathology is long overdue, but before this can be done the following main tasks are still to be performed:

1. Observation, description and classification of mental phenomena.

2. Study of methods of making and recording these observations.

3. Formulation and testing of explanatory hypotheses.

4. Critical scrutiny and clearer definition of our linguistic apparatus, i.e. the descriptive and theoretical terms used by psychopathologists.

5. Analysis of our theoretical conceptions and systems for their logical consistence.

If one is to be strictly scientific and not consider any theory unless it has satisfied all the above criteria, the application of psychopathology to clinical practice will have to wait—perhaps for ever. There is, however, much in existing theories which has clinical validity and can be very helpful in the understanding and treatment of mental illness. Eclecticism based on what is most useful in any theory is the best that can be offered at present to the very wide range of mental illness it is our privilege and responsibility to treat. This does not relieve one of the responsibility of trying to contribute to the elucidation of the above problems.

SECTION 3

NEUROPHYSIOLOGY AND
PSYCHOPHARMACOLOGY

Give an account of **neuronal transmission**

The approaching impulse first causes depolarisation of the cell membrane and concurrently various changes in electric potential take place, including the spike potential of the axon, negative and positive after-potential. These constitute the action potential.

During the action potential the threshold of the neurone to stimulation varies, e.g. a refractory period occurs in association with the spike potential. The nerve cell membrane is normally polarised with positive charges on the outside and negative charges lining the internal surface. During the action potential, this polarity disappears, becoming momentarily reversed. Positive charges from the membrane ahead of and behind the action potential flow into the negative area associated with the action potential, thus decreasing the polarity ahead of the action potential. The series of depolarisation is responsible for circular currents and the self-propagation of the nerve impulse.

In myelinated nerve fibres, circular current flow also occurs, but since myelin is a poor conductor, depolarisation jumps from one node of Ranvier to the next. This jumping of depolarisation is referred to as *saltatory conduction*.

Ionic movement. In nerves, movement of potassium into the cells is associated with transport of sodium outwards. The active movement of sodium against a concentration and electrical gradient sustains the differential surface charges which constitute the resting membrane potential. Depolarisation occurs in association with membrane permeability to sodium ions. This permeability is transient, occurring mainly at the beginning of the action potential. At the peak of the spike potential, the sodium permeability has already returned to the resting situation, allowing repolarisation to ensue. The latter process is also aided by the concomitant changes in potassium permeability.

Define 'all or none' law, rheobase *and* chronaxie

If, in an experimental situation, an axon is stimulated electrically and electrodes are employed for recording purposes at some distance from the stimulating electrodes, the threshold intensity can be measured. The latter signifies the minimum current strength which will just produce an impulse which in turn is indicative of an action potential. Further increases in stimulus intensity will have no effect on the action potential. These data therefore conform to the criteria of the 'all or none' law.

It is further feasible to investigate the relationship between current strength (the stimulus) and the length of time necessary for its application in order to produce a response. The intensity of the stimulating current just sufficient to excite a particular nerve or muscle is the *rheobase*. The term *chronaxie* refers to the length of time a current of twice rheobase strength must be applied to produce a response.

Describe the anatomy and physiology of the **reticular formation**

1. *Anatomy*

The reticular formation begins in the medulla a little above the decussation of the pyramids. It is centrally located and is surrounded by fibre tracts and nuclei associated with the long tract systems, and extends to the pons, midbrain and thalamus. In the thalamus, the relevant anatomical parts are the intralaminar and midline nuclei, including the reticular nucleus. The septal region is often regarded as the rostral end of the reticular formation.

It has numerous afferent and efferent connections, the more important being the principal sensory nuclei, motor cells of the medulla, frontal lobe, sensory and motor cortex, orbital and temporal areas, basal ganglia and cerebellum. The dendrites of a single reticular neurone cover an extensive area, and it is likely that synaptic connection with laterally placed pathways takes place. There is also marked variation in size of these neurones, which permits conduction at short distances. Both slowly and rapidly conducting elements are represented.

2. *Physiology*

Ascending and descending pathways are present, and stimulation experiments have shown inhibitory as well as facilitatory influences to be present. Consequently, the system can influence spinal cord neurones through extrapyramidal projections to the cord. Evoked potentials have also been recorded in the reticular formation following excitation of somatosensory, sympathetic, vagal, auditory, visual and olfactory sources.

Lesions of the midbrain reticular formation cause extreme apathy or somnolence in experimental animals, while electrical stimulation modifies the EEG, producing desynchronisation. It appears that sensory information to the thalamus and further to the cortex is transmitted by ascending pathways in the reticular formation, thus maintaining wakefulness. Studies of single reticular neurones have suggested that they have their own resting rhythm of discharge, often referred to as 'auto-rhythmicity'. But these cells are vulnerable and responsive to a wide variety of incoming nerve impulses.

In addition to sleep/wakefulness the reticular formation is concerned with the following activities: (1) modification and integration of all incoming sensory stimuli; (2) control of visceral and behavioural functions, including an influence on conditioning, through its intimate relationship with the limbic system.

The main function of the reticular formation is to act as a central co-ordinator in the brain, integrating, then modifying incoming stimuli and through its diverse connections controlling and modulating a variety of higher nervous system activities.

Give an account of the **neurophysiology of sleep**

The occurrence of sleep rhythms depends on a balance of activity between the reticular system, cerebral cortex and general sensory input. For example, stimulation of the reticular formation in certain experimental animals produces wakefulness, cortical arousal and activation of the EEG; on the other hand, removal of a cat's cerebral cortex prevents the development of sleep-waking rhythms.

Sleep itself can be divided into several stages, on the basis of EEG changes, alterations in muscle tone and presence or absence of rapid eye movements (REM). REM sleep, although ostensibly a form of deep sleep, often called 'paradoxical sleep', is associated not only with rapid eye movements, but with the EEG of 'lighter sleep', i.e. irregular waves of low voltage.

The following stages of sleep are discernible on EEG recordings:

Stage 1—Drowsiness, eyes being closed. Alpha rhythm is still present, and disappears on opening the eyes.

Stage 2—Alpha rhythm gives way to flatter, slower waves as drowsiness progresses to sleep. Sleep is still light and any novel stimulus can cause alpha rhythm to reappear.

Stage 3—EEG shows slower waves which are irregular. Bursts of faster waves ('sleep spindles') occur in this stage of deeper sleep. Also, appropriate external stimuli may produce a wave configuration called the K complex. The latter consists of a small sharp wave followed by one or more larger slow waves, followed by faster waves.

Stage 4—High-voltage slow waves (1 to 2 per sec.). K complexes still obtainable.

Stage 5—High-voltage slow waves, as in Stage 4. K complexes do not appear.

During a night's sleep, shifts occur between the various stages. A normal person has several periods of deep sleep during the night, more commonly in the early period of sleep. It is during stages of deep sleep that the features associated with REM (or 'paradoxical') sleep occur, including dreams.

'Orthodox' sleep is characterised by:

1. Large slow waves on the EEG.
2. Eyes are relatively immobile.
3. Some muscles, e.g. of the throat, are tense.
4. Heart is regular.

'Paradoxical' sleep is characterised by:

1. Small irregular waves.
2. Rapid eye movements.
3. Throat muscles are relaxed.
4. Heart tends to be irregular.

Patients with narcolepsy develop paradoxical sleep with great facility.

Barbiturates and amphetamines reduce the amount of REM sleep; and when barbiturate hypnotics are withdrawn, the sleep rhythm does not return to normal for about five weeks.

Most of the facts about the neurophysiological basis of sleep have been obtained from animal experiments, especially with cats. From such sources it has been shown that REM (paradoxical) sleep is associated with hindbrain activity; and it is already known that in this part of the brain (midbrain, pons and medulla in humans) is located the major part of the reticular activating system. Cells of the visual cortex of cats are more active, on the other hand, during orthodox ('forebrain', 'cortical') sleep.

Describe the **thalamic nuclei** *and the functions of the* **thalamus**

There are several dozen thalamic 'nuclei', which are grouped regionally:

1. *Anterior*

This is separated from the rest of the thalamus by the limbs of the internal medullary lamina. It receives fibres from the mammillary bodies via the mammillothalamic tract and projects to the cingulate cortex.

2. *Lateral*

Lies anterior to the pulvinar between the internal and external medullary lamina.

(a) Anterior ventral, with connections with the corpus striatum.

(b) Lateral ventral, which receives fibres from the superior cerebellar peduncle and projects to the premotor and motor cortex.

(c) Posterior ventral, receives fibres from the medial lemniscus, spinothalamic and trigeminal tracts, and projects to the sensory cortex.

(d) Dorsolateral and posterolateral nuclei receive fibres from other thalamic nuclei and project to the parietal cortex.

(e) Reticular nucleus, lies between the internal capsule and the external medullary lamina and is continuous with the *zona incerta*.

3. *Posterior*

(*a*) Pulvinar, receives fibres from the other thalamic nuclei and geniculate bodies, and projects to the posterior parts of the parietal and temporal lobes.

(*b*) Medial geniculate body, receives auditory fibres from the lateral lemniscus and inferior quadrigeminal body and projects via the auditory radiation to the temporal cortex.

(*c*) Lateral geniculate body, receives optic tract fibres and projects via the optic (geniculocalcarine) radiation to the visual (calcarine) cortex.

4. *Medial*

Lies between nuclei of midline and internal medullary lamina.

(*a*) Dorsal medial has connections with other thalamic nuclei and hypothalamus, and projects to the frontal cortex.

(*b*) Centrum medianum, with thalamic and corpus striatal connections.

5. *Midline*

These nuclei are situated beneath the lining of the third ventricle, and have connections with the hypothalamus, periaqueductal region and anterior rhinencephalon.

In summary, the thalamic nuclei have close subcortical connections, e.g. to other parts of the thalamus, hypothalamus, basal ganglia and subthalamus, and therefore have some degree of local regulating activity and control. The thalamus also houses many relay stations to sensory cortex as well as to and from association cortex. It is thought that the thalamus may be an important centre for perception of some sensory modalities, being complemented by the sensory cortex, which presumably has a higher but similar function in perception.

There is some evidence that the reticular formation has rostral extensions in the thalamus. Stimulation of the midline nuclei of the thalamus (which have connections with midbrain reticular formation, limbic system and sensory collaterals) has an effect on the resting EEG, recorded from the cortex. It is likely that impulses from the reticular system of the thalamus play an important role in regulating the electrical activity of the cortex. However, thalamo-cortical connections are not all in the one direction, and it is probable that 'feed-back' takes place.

There are two important clinical applications of thalamic anatomy. A lesion in the thalamus, often cerebrovascular but occasionally neoplastic, may cause the 'thalamic syndrome' which is characterised by hemianaesthesia followed by unpleasant sensations. In the operation of prefrontal leucotomy, thalamo-frontal connections are interrupted; a similar effect can be obtained by placing a lesion in the dorsomedial nucleus of the thalamus.

Give an account of the hypothalamus

The hypothalamus lies ventral to the thalamus, forming the floor and part of the walls of the third ventricle; it comprises the following parts: mammillary bodies, tuber cinereum, infundibulum and optic chiasma. The infundibulum links the hypothalamus to the posterior lobe of the pituitary.

The nuclei of the hypothalamus can be divided as follows:

1. Anterior group—paraventricular and supraoptic nuclei; the latter are connected to the pituitary by the supraoptico-hypophyseal tract.
2. Lateral.
3. Middle—dorsomedial and ventromedial nuclei.
4. Posterior—lie anterior to the mammillary bodies; also includes the nuclei of the mammillary bodies.

The main connections of the hypothalamus are:

1. *Afferent*
   (*a*) Medial forebrain bundle bringing impulses from the frontal lobe.
   (*b*) Fibres from thalamus.
   (*c*) Fornix, which arises in the hippocampus and terminates in the mammillary bodies.
   (*d*) Stria terminalis (from amygdala to preoptic region).

2. *Efferent*
   (*a*) Mammillo-thalamic tract—to cingulate cortex.
   (*b*) Fibres in medial forebrain bundle running to lower centres.

(c) Two tracts to the pituitary.

(d) Projections to cortex.

(e) Periventricular fibres to lower levels.

Their functions are diverse: (1) Control of body temperature; lesions of the hypothalamus may lead to loss of control, with fluctuations related to the environment. The anterior part is concerned with heat loss mechanisms whereas heat production and conservation resides in the posterior region. (2) Control of hunger and thirst, as well as to some extent sexual drive. (3) In animals, lesions may produce starvation, or more medially, obesity. By placing electrodes in different parts of the hypothalamus of experimental animals, not only can discrete lesions be placed and their effects observed, but the effect of stimulation can also be examined. Centres in the lateral hypothalamus are concerned with reinforcement of behaviour; e.g. reward effects have been obtained by stimulation of the posterior part of the lateral hypothalamus (corresponding to part of the medial forebrain bundle), and a negative (aversive) area has also been demonstrated. Autonomic activity can be produced by electric stimulation, while vague emotional changes have been experienced during stimulation in patients undergoing stereotaxic techniques.

The most important function of the hypothalamus is probably integrative, acting in association with the forebrain, brain stem and limbic system. It thus plays an important role in the regulation of sleep and waking as well as of emotional, autonomic and motor activities.

Lesions of the hypothalamus in man may lead to diabetes insipidus, obesity, disturbances of sleep, feeding, autonomic activity and temperature control.

Discuss the **limbic system**

The limbic system consists of several structures, including cortical and subcortical grey matter as well as short and long fibre tracts, and is situated around the corpus callosum and brain stem close to the medial parts of the cerebral hemisphere. Some of these structures were previously regarded as subserving only olfactory functions, on account of their location in the rhinencephalon. Papez suggested that the limbic system provided a functional circuit concerned with the emotions, and that the structures constituting the limbic system provided pathways to and from the hippocampus.

The limbic system can be divided into two groups:

1. The *'inner ring'*—amygdala, hippocampus, septal area, fornix, stria terminalis and medial forebrain bundle.

2. The *'outer ring'*—cingulum, hippocampus and tracts to the anterior cortex.

It has been suggested that the inner ring deals with fast reflexes via the brain stem, while the outer ring evaluates the internal environment and deals with 'extra-limbic' cortex as well as with the inner limbic ring.

The following are the more important connections of the limbic system:

1. The fornix—leads from hippocampus to mammillary body.

2. Mammillo-thalamic tract—projects from mammillary body to anterior thalamus, and thence to the cingular cortex.

3. Cingulum—from cingular cortex to hippocampus.

4. Medial forebrain bundle—carries afferent and efferent pathways to and from the limbic system connecting with the frontal lobe, hypothalamus and reticular formation.

5. Stria terminalis—from amygdala to hypothalamus.

6. Stria medullaris and the Meynert bundle, from amygdala to the habenular nuclei.

The limbic system, through its widespread connections, has an integrative function, as does also the hypothalamus, with which it is intimately connected.

Ablation studies in animals have shown that damage to the limbic system leads to changes in emotion and in motor activity. However, there are individual differences, e.g. Rhesus monkeys are made tame, whereas cats are rendered aggressive. Conditioning experiments in animals indicate that various types of learned behaviour are affected by lesions of the limbic system; in particular the acquisition of conditioned avoidance responses is interfered with, especially with lesions of the amygdala and mammillary bodies. Some forms of conditioning in animals are associated with changes in the EEG of the hippocampus. Learning, and consequently memory, is thus dependent on the intact limbic system. Patients with temporal lobe epilepsy may have not only episodic emotional disturbances, but also memory disturbances, e.g. *déjà vu, jamais vu* and panoramic memory. Bilateral temporal lobectomy in such patients often leads to difficulties in learning ability, especially auditory verbal learning. The classical studies of Penfield have demonstrated how stimulation of the temporal lobe at operation may produce emotional and memory experiences. Bilateral lesions of the hippocampus in man can lead to memory difficulties; the Korsakow syndrome in chronic alcoholics tends to be associated with pathology in the region of the mammillary bodies. It is thought that the limbic system plays an essential part in the 'second stage of memory', i.e. after sensory impulses have led to actual perception. The present experience is then assessed in the light of the emotional state, state of consciousness and previous memories. The theory goes that only then do permanent molecular changes occur (involving DNA and RNA) leading to the laying down of a more permanent memory, involving other areas of the brain, in addition to the limbic system. The hippocampus is necessary for the retention of long-term memory.

The limbic system has in the past been called the 'visceral brain' or thymencephalon, in that its functions are concerned with the interpretation of experience in terms of feeling and emotion rather than intellect. Limbic system connections with the hypothalamus and brain stem allow modulation of information from the internal environment, while widespread connections with cortex and reticular formation facilitate scanning of perceptual activity and somatic stimuli.

Discuss **physiological measures of anxiety**

The bodily manifestations (and consequently symptoms) of anxiety are protean and are reflected by physiological changes in many body systems.

Many such changes are measurable and include the following:

1. Blood flow through various regions of the body, e.g. finger tip blood flow mirrors skin blood flow, and forearm blood flow reflects muscle blood flow.

2. Other cardiovascular measures, e.g. pulse rate and blood pressure.

3. Size of pupils.

4. Salivary secretion.

5. Respiratory movements and efficiency.

6. Electromyography which enables detailed study of electrical activity in accessible muscles.

7. Electroencephalogram. (See Section 4.)   In general, EEG changes in patients with anxiety are non-specific and variable.

8. Sweat gland activity of the palms, variations in which lead to consequent changes in the electrical resistance (*conductance*) of the skin.   Various stimuli, e.g. auditory and tactile, produce alterations in skin resistance which has been termed galvanic skin response (GSR) or psychogalvanic reflex (PGR).

Many physiological measures are elevated in anxious patients, e.g. respiration is more rapid and often less efficient; skin conductance is raised in association with increased palmar sweating; pulse rate, forearm blood flow and blood presure is raised.

These measures are useful in monitoring the level of anxiety in patients compared with normals.   It has been found that anxious patients continue to demonstrate enhanced physiological activity long after the cessation of stimulation, while normal subjects adjust more quickly as reflected in a more rapid return to resting levels.   Similarly, normal subjects *habituate* more readily than anxious patients.   This means that on repetitive stimulation they show progressively weaker responses compared with anxious patients, who show impaired habituation with skin conductance and on EEG.

Some of the physiological measures which are altered in states of anxiety are also influenced by other emotional states, e.g. rage.

In fact, none of the above mentioned measures is specific for anxiety.   Therefore in recent years the *concept of 'arousal'* has gained adherents.

What is meant by **arousal**?

This concept has been developed to explain the relationship between emotional state and corresponding physiological measures (see preceding question).

Arousal refers to a spectrum of activity ranging from sleep to alertness.   Along this continuum, levels of behavioural arousal

C

are associated with corresponding physiological measures. High levels of arousal are associated with feelings of being on edge and with other expressions of anxiety. Higher levels are accompanied by anger and similar feelings. Extreme emotional states, such as terror and abnormal euphoria, are regarded in this concept, as reflecting extremely high levels of arousal.

Although the physiological correlates of arousal with a particular emotional state tend to be consistent in an individual, these physiological measures vary enormously among individuals. These measurements are therefore more useful in monitoring changes in one individual than in studying comparisons between groups of patients.

Comment on **specificity of physiological response**

Individuals vary in their bodily reactions to stimulation but for any one individual, the physiological responses for any specific stimulation are remarkably consistent. These patterns depend not only on factors based on the individual's physiological make-up, but also on factors to do with the stimulus or *response specificity*. This has some application in the understanding of *psychosomatic disorders* and *symptom specificity* in that a somatic symptom may depend on a particular physiological response which may be provoked by some form of stress.

What are the **sources of energy** *for the central nervous system?*

Fat, carbohydrates and proteins, in the form of foodstuffs, ultimately undergo various catabolic reactions. Firstly, fat, carbohydrate and protein molecules are broken down to fatty acids, glycerol, hexoses and amino acids. Secondly, each of these substances is connected into a carboxylic acid, releasing about one-third of the total energy produced. The carboxylic acids concerned are acetic acid, α-ketoglutaric acid and oxaloacetic acid. These acids are then oxidised in the third phase, which is the citric acid cycle, during which the remaining two-thirds of the energy is liberated. During these oxidations, hydrogen atoms become free and convert nicotinamide or flavoprotein coenzymes to their reduced forms; reoxidation of the latter by oxygen requires a chain of enzymatic processes, often called 'the respiratory chain'. During its operation, adenosine diphosphate (ADP) is converted to adenosine triphosphate (ATP). Energy is stored and ultimately utilised, by means of the phosphate linkages ('energy bonds') of ATP.

In CNS metabolism, glucose is the principal source of energy. Glucose is catabolised to two molecules of pyruvic acid, by means of the process of glycolysis. The latter can occur aerobically or anaerobically. In anaerobic glycolysis, the pyruvate is converted to lactic acid, with the ultimate production of two molecules of ATP from every one molecule of glucose. When the glycolysis takes place aerobically, pyruvic acid can be converted to an activated form of acetic acid, viz. acetylcoenzyme A. The latter can then enter the carboxylic (Krebs) cycle; each acetyl molecule dealt with in this way produces two molecules of carbon dioxide, liberating eight atoms of hydrogen. The hydrogen atoms are utilised in the reduction of nicotinamide or flavoprotein coenzymes, which can subsequently be oxidised, and further reduced, by means of the respiratory chain. Each cycle yields 4 molecules of water and 12 molecules of ATP. The total aerobic breakdown of one glucose molecule produces 38 molecules of ATP.

How is **acetylcholine** *produced, and what are its functions?*

Free choline and activated acetate (acetylcoenzyme A) combine, in the presence of choline acetylase and, utilising energy from ATP, form acetylcholine. The activated acetate is obtained from glucose metabolism, but may also derive from the metabolism of amino acids, and fatty acids.

It is thought that acetylcholine is synthesised in the body of cholinergic neurones, being subsequently carried peripherally. It is held, in a bound inactivated form, in small vesicles which become concentrated at the synaptic knob. Collision between a vesicle and the presynaptic membrane causes acetylcholine to be released. When the membrane is depolarised by a nerve impulse, many collisions occur, with the release of free acetylcholine. The latter then travels across the synapse. The enzyme acetylcholinesterase destroys free acetylcholine.

Acetylcholine has an important role as a transmitter substance, association with the following:

1. Motor end-plate.
2. Pre-ganglionic parasympathetic fibres.
3. Post-ganglionic parasympathetic fibres.

4. Pre-ganglionic sympathetic fibres.

Acetylcholine tends to act, when released from vagal cardiac fibres, as an inhibitor.

What are the catecholamines?

The catecholamines include adrenaline, noradrenaline and dopamine. The main route of biosynthesis of these substances is as follows:

1. Phenylalanine is converted to tyrosine; enzyme concerned is phenylalanine hydroxylase.

2. Tyrosine is converted to dihydroxyphenylalanine (DOPA) which becomes dihydroxyphenylethylamine (DOPAMINE) under the influence of DOPA decarboxylase.

3. Dopamine is converted to noradrenaline, the action being mediated by dopamine oxidase.

4. Adrenaline is obtained from noradrenaline by the action of phenylethanolamine N-methyl transferase.

The highest concentration of noradrenaline is in the hypo-thalamus, whereas adrenaline is found mainly in the adrenal medulla, with a low concentration in the brain. Dopamine is most concentrated in the caudate and lentiform nuclei. Reduced levels have been found in Parkinsonism, hence L-dopa has been used in its treatment.

Noradrenaline functions mainly as a transmitter substance in the peripheral sympathetic system. The role of this and of the other catechol amines in the CNS is still not clear. Noradrenaline is stored, in sympathetic fibres, in intraneuronal granules; there are thought to be two metabolic pools which exist in dynamic equilibrium. One is labile and may be released by nerve stimuli or by sympathomimetic drugs, e.g. amphetamines; the other, which presumably functions as a storage reservoir, can be released by reserpine. The brain concentration of noradrenaline is increased by drugs which inhibit monoamine oxidase. It is probable that noradrenaline is synthesised and stored at its site of action, the adrenergic axon. The amount of noradrenaline present in auto-nomic nerves is proportional to the number of adrenergic fibres.

Destruction of noradrenaline
Once released, noradrenaline is destroyed in one of several ways.

Some of it is removed by monoamine oxidase (MAO) and converted to dihydroxymandelic acid. Most of it is converted to normetradrenaline by catechol-O-methyl transferase (COMT). The intermediary metabolites, normetradrenaline and dihydroxymandelic acid, can be further acted upon by MAO and COMT respectively, with the production of vanillylmandelic acid (VMA) which is excreted. It is believed that some noradrenaline is inactivated at the receptor site, without passage to the blood stream and urinary excretion. It is most likely that O-methylation is a far commoner process of elimination of noradrenaline than monoamine oxidation. It is still uncertain whether the catechol amines and serotonin act separately as transmitters, or whether they act as modulators or regulators of synaptic transmission mediated by a transmitter such as acetylcholine.

What is the origin, function and fate of **Serotonin?**

Serotonin (5-hydroxytryptamine) is present in many tissues of the body; the highest concentrations are found in the intestinal mucosa, but it is also found in blood platelets, spleen and CNS. Its distribution and concentration in the brain is similar to that of noradrenaline, i.e. mainly in hypothalamus and adjacent grey matter. The distribution of 5-hydroxytryptophan decarboxylase parallels that of serotonin; thus it is probable that serotonin can be synthesised in the CNS. There is some evidence to suggest that this decarboxylase requires the presence of pyridoxal phosphate.

Tryptophan is converted to 5-hydroxytryptophan (5HTP). The latter is acted upon by 5HTP decarboxylase to produce 5-hydroxytryptamine (5HT or serotonin).

Reserpine is capable of releasing 5HT from the gut, platelets and brain.

Serotonin is oxidised by monoamine oxidase, first to aldehyde and then to 5-hydroxyindole acetic acid (5HIAA) which is excreted in the urine. This metabolic pathway is probably not unique in the destruction of 5HT, since when 5HT is injected, only about one-third can be recovered as urinary 5HIAA.

Although levels of 5HT are often increased by the action of monoamine oxidase inhibiting drugs, and the latter are at times able to produce antidepressant changes in patients, the physiological role of serotonin remains uncertain. One view is that it acts, as does acetylcholine and noradrenaline, as a neurohumoral transmitter at synapses. On the other hand, it is suggested that it acts as one of the regulators and controllers of synaptic transmission, where the basic transmitter is another substance, e.g. acetylcholine.

What is the association between **cybernetics** *and psychiatry?*

The word 'cybernetics' was introduced by Wiener in 1948 from the Greek word for a steersman, and has been defined as that branch of science which studies, in complex mechanisms, *the lines of communication*, which may be established between part and part, the *information* which may be transmitted along them, the *control* which each part thereby establishes over the other, and the *co-ordination* which is thereby achieved. The Latinised version of cybernetics is 'governor', which was the name given to Watt's self-correcting device for his steam engine and one of the earliest examples of regulation in mechanical invention. Prior to this application, machines were controlled by the human brain through a system of levers; later, energy was stored in the machine as in the clock-spring; later still, as in Watt's steam engine, the machine became capable of transforming energy and to a certain extent controlling the output.

The subject is sprinkled with a number of definitions derived from communication theory, and as these have close analogy with brain function, the relationship between cybernetics and psychiatry has been explored and developed. Some of these concepts are control, information, storage of information, control by pattern, goal-seeking behaviour, stability, feedback both negative and positive and circulating processes. The concept of a second-order feedback with step functions has been used to explain learning and adaptation in the human organism, and the brain function analogy of the machine has been used to include definitions of induction, deduction, prediction, decision-making, trial and error, selection and also dreaming. The whole subject is a complex one and for a full understanding of it a knowledge of physics and mathematics is becoming increasingly important. The analogy is probably the most sophisticated one that has yet been developed to explain brain function in higher animals, including man, and much more evidence is likely to be forthcoming in the future.

At the same time, analogies are not new and all-embracing ones are suspect. Cybernetics does convey an air of precision which because of its veneer of mathematical certainty will find adherents and even fanatical devotees. The models used are physical, and while illustrating possible methods of storing information in the brain and of learning, they are seriously deficient in other biological and human functions. The human brain is not nearly as sensitive as the machine to trauma and has considerable compensatory powers when deprived of large areas either through disease or surgery. It also has emotional functions which are lacking in the machine. It is possible to say that the machine looks 'puzzled' or 'angry', but these are illusions, for feeling has not yet reached the machine.

What are the **tranquillisers** *and how are they classified?*

They have a sedative effect without lowering the level of consciousness. They can be classified as follows :

1. Major tranquillisers
   (*a*) Phenothiazines;
   (*b*) Reserpine;
   (*c*) Butyrophenones;
   (*d*) Diphenobutopiperidines, e.g. pimozide;
   (*e*) Thioxanthenes, e.g. depixol.
2. Minor tranquillisers
   (*a*) Benzdiazepines, e.g. chlordiazepoxide and diazepam;
   (*b*) Meprobamate;
   (*c*) Diphenylmethane derivatives, e.g. hydroxyzine and benactyzine;
   (*d*) Diphenylbutylpiperidine, e.g. pimozide;
   (*e*) Thioxanthenes, e.g. flupenthixol.

Give an account of the **phenothiazines,** *including their classification, action, uses and side-effects*

A. The phenothiazines can be *classified* as follows:
   1. 3-carbon aliphatic side-chain, e.g. chlorpromazine, promazine.
   2. Piperidine side-chain, e.g. thioridazine, mepazine.
   3. Piperazine side-chain, e.g. trifluoperazine, prochlorperazine.

B. *Actions* of the phenothiazines:

Area of activity is subcortical; there is evidence that Chlorpromazine acts on the reticular formation, hypothalamus and electrical phenomena have been evoked in the amygdala. Chlorpromazine (i) interferes with certain enzymes, and in animals acts on ATP metabolism in the brain; (ii) acts as a sympatholytic antihistamine and blocks the alerting effect of biogenic amines. (iii) produces increase in weight mainly by water retention and has a mild diabetogenic action.

C. *Uses* of the phenothiazines:

1. Schizophrenia: chlorpromazine is more effective when the patient is agitated or restless. In the withdrawn apathetic schizophrenic, one of the piperazine group is to be preferred. Fluphenazine decanoate is an injectable long-acting phenothiazine which may be useful when treating chronic schizophrenics who are reluctant to take tablets.
2. Mania and hypomania.
3. Hyperactivity associated with organic states, such as delirium, confusional states and dementia, and post-leucotomy restlessness or aggressive tendencies.
4. Alcoholism and drug addiction in the phase of withdrawal, e.g. delirium tremens in an alcoholic.
5. Post-operative and puerperal psychoses.
6. Hyperemesis gravidarum.
7. Anorexia nervosa.
8. Potentiation of the effect of a hypnotic or analgesic.

D. *Toxic effects:*

1. Jaundice—of obstructive type, and may resemble infective hepatitis.
2. Dermatitis, photosensitivity.
3. Leucopenia, may be presenting as a pyrexia.
4. Lactation.
5. Melanosis (pigmentation).
   These toxic effects are more or less specific to chlorpromazine. General side-effects of any phenothiazine include:
6. Hypotension, especially in the elderly.
7. Extrapyramidal effects.—These are more commonly seen

in therapy with the piperazine group, and consist of (i) Parkinsonism, with tremor and rigidity; (ii) akathisia (extreme restlessness); (iii) dystonic or dyskinetic reactions —these take the form of involuntary movements affecting the neck, face, lips, tongue, trunk or upper limbs. In brain-damaged or post-leucotomy patients medicated with large doses of phenothiazines over a prolonged period, such dyskinesias may become permanent and are called *tardive dyskinesia*.

How are toxic effects *managed?*

In the more severe type of toxic effect, viz. leucopenia or jaundice, the drug must be stopped. Reduction of the dosage may well suffice in control of the other side-effects. Extrapyramidal side-effects can be specifically dealt with by means of one of the anti-Parkinsonian drugs, e.g. benzhexol (Artane), benztropine (Cogentin) or orphenadrine (Disipal). On the occurrence of a severe dystonic reaction, parenteral administration of promethazine (Phenergan) or benztropine is indicated. Thiopropazate (Dartalan) and tetrabenazine (Nitoman) are also useful in tardive dyskinesia.

Write a note on reserpine

This is one of the alkaloids of Rauwolfia serpentina, an Indian shrub which was used for centuries as a medicament, including use in treatment of mental illness. Reserpine liberates serotonin and catechol amines from nervous tissues; it releases serotonin from platelets and intestine, as well as from the brain and its action is primarily as an inhibitor of cortical activity, although its site of action is probably mainly subcortical, as in the case of the phenothiazines.

Uses. As an alternative to other major tranquillisers in the treatment of schizophrenia.

Side-effects. (1) Depression, especially in the susceptible patient receiving the drug over a prolonged period, e.g. in the management of hypertension. The depression often remains after the drug is stopped. (2) Parkinsonism. (3) Hypotension.

What are the butyrophenones?

This group of drugs is chemically related to gamma-amino

butyric acid (GABA), which is a normally occurring brain constituent. Activity and site of action are similar to those of the phenothiazines, excepting negligible sympatholytic (adrenolytic) activity and no effect on the blood pressure.

Examples. Haloperidol, Triperidol.

Uses. Similar to those of the phenothiazines, but especially: (1) As an alternative to phenothiazines in treatment of schizophrenia and organic psychoses. (2) Treatment of mania and hypomania. It is increasingly held that Haloperidol is the drug of choice in these conditions. (3) Alcoholism—in delirium tremens.

Side-effects. Mainly extrapyramidal, viz. Parkinsonism, akathisia, dyskinesias.

Write a note on the **benzdiazepines**

This group of drugs consists of substances such as chlordiazepoxide and diazepam (Librium and Valium respectively) which are minor tranquillisers. They are often referred to as 'anxiolytics', since their main action is to reduce anxiety and tension.

Drugs in this group experimentally increase the threshold to electrically induced convulsions. They thus have a mild anticonvulsant action and like barbiturates produce some fast activity on the EEG.

Uses. (1) Reduction of anxiety in neurotic illnesses and psychosomatic disorders. (2) Adjunct to antidepressants in neurotic depression. (3) Adjunct to established anticonvulsants in the treatment of epilepsy. (4) Delirium tremens, used intravenously.

Toxic effects. (1) Addiction. (2) Ataxia. (3) Drowsiness.

What is the action and use of **meprobamate?**

It is related chemically to the muscle relaxant, mephenesin, and has similar properties in addition to mild tranquillising effects. Of limited use in the treatment (usually in general practice) of neurosis.

Relatively free of side-effects, but cases of addiction have been reported, with delirium tremens on withdrawal of the drug.

Describe the action and uses of the **amphetamines**

The amphetamines are sympathomimetic amines related to

adrenaline and ephedrine. In excessive dosage they lead to wakefulness.

In animals, the behavioural arousal which is produced by amphetamines is accompanied by desynchronisation of the EEG. In man, effects similar to caffeine and adrenaline, viz. a shift to faster frequencies, is produced only on high dosage. The barbiturated fast EEG is neutralised.

Uses. (1) Depression in old people or those with serious physical illnesses, where the hypotensive side-effects of antidepressant drugs are to be avoided. (2) Narcolepsy. (3) Behaviour disorders in childhood, including hyperkinetic brain-damaged children. (4) As anticonvulsant, e.g. in petit mal. (5) Abreaction—given intravenously on its own, or together with pentothal. (6) Impotence in middle age.

Give an account of the classification, mode of action, uses and side-effects of the **antidepressant drugs**

A. *Classification:*
 The antidepressant drugs are divided into two main groups:

1. Monoamine oxidase inhibitors (MAOI), e.g. phenelzine (Nardil), isocarboxazid (Marplan), iproniazid (Marsilid) and tranylcypromine (Parnate).
2. Tricyclic compounds, e.g. imipramine (Tofranil), dothiepin (Prothiaden), amitriptyline, nortriptyline and protriptyline; dibenzepin.
3. Tetracyclic-maprotiline (Ludiomil).

B. *Action:*

1. MAOI group. Drugs in this group inhibit monoamine oxidase, which is thought to play a part in the metabolism of serotonin and the catechol amines. Animals given MAOI become excited and increased brain levels of noradrenaline and serotonin are subsequently found. The precursor of serotonin, 5-hydroxytryptophan, and the precursor of catechol amines, dihydroxyphenylalanine (DOPA), both have excitatory effects which can be potentiated by MAOI. The sedation and ptosis in mice, brought about by reserpine, can be blocked by previous administration of MAOI.

Following administration of MAOI, a maximal concentration of serotonin is found in the brain after four weeks. Consequently, on theoretical grounds at least, a period of four weeks would seem to be a maximum trial period for a MAOI drug. REM sleep is abolished but only after three weeks and this may be related to its pharmacological action on the brain. However, there are still many unknown facts about normal amine metabolism, and the concentration of brain amines does not necessarily mirror the degree of MAO inhibition; and the latter is not consistently related to relief of depression.

2. Tricyclic group. Drugs in this group do not inhibit monoamine oxidase, although they produce an increase in free monoamines in the nervous tissues of animals. They also depress REM sleep but not so markedly as the MAOI drugs. Tricyclic drugs potentiate both the effects of amphetamines, as well as sympathetic responses generally and the effects of administered noradrenaline. It is thought that they act by inhibiting cellular uptake and inactivation of noradrenaline. Reserpine-induced sedation in animals can be prevented by tricyclic drugs.

C. *Uses:*

Either group of antidepressant drugs can be used in the treatment of a depressive illness of any type; there is some evidence to suggest that the tricyclic group are more effective than the MAOI in psychotic (endogenous) types of depression, whereas the MAOI have their place in the treatment of neurotic depressions and mixed types of neurosis, e.g. phobic anxiety states with depressive features. In such conditions, the MAOI can be combined with a minor tranquilliser, e.g. one of the benzdiazepine group. The tricyclic antidepressants are generally safer to use than the MAOI. 'Combined antidepressants' are sometimes advocated in the treatment of resistant depressions, i.e. tricyclic+MAOI drugs given together. This can sometimes lead to toxic effects and is normally practised only under hospital supervision. Antidepressant drugs are used, as well as in depressive illnesses and some neuroses, in:

1. Some cases of schizo-affective illness, used in combination with a major tranquilliser.
2. Some patients with pain, e.g. atypical facial pain.

D. *Side-effects:*

1. MAOI

   (a) Hypertensive crises, headaches: these may be precipitated by certain foodstuffs (cheese containing high concentration of tyramine, broad beans which contain DOPA, beef extracts and yeast), alcohol, narcotic drugs, e.g. pethidine, sympathomimetic amines, e.g. amphetamines, other antidepressant drugs, e.g. tricyclics. Tranylcypromine (Parnate) is the MAOI most likely to be associated with this side-effect. (Several cases of subarachnoid haemorrhage have been reported.)
   (b) Hypotension.
   (c) Liver damage—risk is highest with iproniazid.
   (d) Rashes or reactivation of eczema.
   (e) Danger of apnoea after anaesthetic procedures, e.g. for operations or ECT since serum pseudo-cholinesterase is sometimes inhibited thus prolonging the effect of relaxants.
   (f) Potentiation of insulin-induced hypoglycaemia.

2. Tricyclic

   (a) Hypotension—giddiness, occasionally collapse.
   (b) Sweating, tachycardia.
   (c) Atropine-like effects, viz. dryness of mouth, constipation, difficulty in visual accommodation, urinary retention (mainly in the male). Should not be given to patient with glaucoma.
   (d) Occasional cardiac irregularities, with an abnormal ECG.
   (e) Interference with the action of hypotensive drugs, often reducing their efficiency.

Describe the uses, as well as the biochemical, pharmacological and toxic effects of **lithium preparations**

Lithium, the lightest in weight of all solids, was first isolated in

1855 and has been used in various manufacturing processes, including dehumidifying agents, ceramics and hydrogen bombs. It was first used in medicine in the treatment of gout, and as a vehicle for bromide was an early form of sedative. Cade in Australia introduced lithium salts, in 1949, into psychiatric practice in the treatment of mania. With the recent revival of interest in these compounds, it has been shown that their main use lies in the prevention of recurrence of attacks in manic-depressives, though it is doubtful if they are effective in the treatment of depression. Lithium carbonate is the usual pre-scribed form, tablets as well as sustained release preparations being available. In Scandinavia, the citrate is also used. (See Section 9, Affective Disorders, for further details about administration.) Lithium does not seem to produce any effects when given to normal individuals. Excretion varies according to whether the patient is manic or depressed, the manic patient tending to retain lithium longer and being able to tolerate higher doses. It is excreted almost entirely by the kidneys, 50 per cent every 24 hours, and resembles sodium in its electrolytic properties, and is capable of displacing it from cells. Sodium restriction in the diet therefore encourages lithium retention in the body. The sodium diuresis provoked by lithium leads to compensatory hormonal changes, e.g. initial increase in aldosterone excretion. The effects of lithium on water and electrolyte metabolism are complex and their significance, for example, on magnesium and calcium metabolism still remains unclear.

Amine metabolism is also affected by lithium. It has been shown to facilitate re-uptake of noradrenaline by presynaptic neurones and it has been suggested that lithium reduces the amount of noradrenaline available for action as a transmitter for central adrenergic activity. Serotonin turnover may also be influenced.

Toxic effects. These increase in number and severity as blood and tissue levels of lithium rise. There is marked variation among individuals in vulnerability to side-effects. Kidney disease or restriction of sodium in the diet will tend to accentuate lithium levels and therefore the occurrence of toxicity.

Side-effects are:

1. Gastro-intestinal: Anorexia, dry mouth, metallic taste, diarrhoea, nausea, vomiting.
2. Neuromuscular: Weakness, muscle irritability, tremor.
3. CNS: Skin anaesthesia, dysarthria, ataxia, dizziness, incontinence, epileptic fits, EEG changes.
4. CVS: Pulse irregularities, fall in blood pressure.
5. Miscellaneous: Polyuria and thirst, enlargement of thyroid gland (goitre), hypothyroidism.

SECTION 4

THE EEG IN PSYCHIATRY

Describe the **frequency bands** *in the electroencephalogram (EEG)*

The EEG records and emphasises spike potentials picked up by scalp electrodes and the electrical patterns are finally manifested on the EEG as waves. The frequencies of these waves are divided for convenience into various bands named after letters of the Greek alphabet and measured as cycles per second. (1) Alpha band, rhythm or activity: from 8 to 13 c./s. This is seen in the parieto-occipital areas in a normal EEG and is blocked by eye opening or by active mental processes. (2) Beta band: faster than 13 c./s., usually in the range 14 to 30 c./s. It is seen in many normal EEGs and is commoner in older subjects. Barbiturates may also increase the amount of fast activity. (3) Theta activity: 4 to 7 c./s.: frequently seen in young people and in immature personalities, such as psychopaths. Widespread theta activity is abnormal. (4) Delta: this refers to frequencies below 4 c./s. and is usually abnormal when seen on the EEG of an alert adult subject. Slow waves, i.e. in the theta and delta bands, are more likely to be abnormal the greater the voltage they attain.

Describe a **child's EEG**

In the first few months of life the EEG tends to be of relatively low voltage and contains much slow activity in the theta and delta bands. By the age of 2 years alpha rhythm has commenced and slow activity is now represented by well-formed theta waves. The EEGs of children from 2 to 12 years tend to be polyrhythmic and with increasing age the child's EEG shows a tendency for the various wave forms to become situated posteriorly. With the approach of puberty the alpha activity tends to displace the slower theta rhythms, which may persist into adolescence and are also seen in immature adults, in epileptics and schizophrenics.

What are **provocation techniques?**

These refer to various manoeuvres which potentiate an EEG abnormality which is not obvious on a routine record.

1. Hyperventilation. Over-breathing tends to exaggerate EEG abnormalities, especially of the epileptic variety. In a normal individual, rapid over-breathing leads to slow-wave abnormalities over the frontal leads and is more marked in children than in adults. Some epileptic patients produce a normal, or border-line abnormal EEG, but after hyperventilation definite epileptic EEG manifestations are often evoked, e.g. the spike and wave abnormality which is characteristic of petit mal.

2. Hypoglycaemia. This can be produced by fasting or by injection of tolbutamide. It makes the EEG record more sensitive to hyperventilation.

3. Photic stimulation. It is well established that major or minor epileptic fits may be provoked by a rhythmically flashing light, consequently photic stimulation may be employed as a provocation technique. Spikes may occur at the same frequency as the flashing light or there may be evoked widespread repetitive spike and wave discharges. Photic stimulation may produce associated clinical phenomena such as jerkings or disturbances of consciousness.

4. Analeptic drugs. Leptazol and bemegride activate the EEGs of suspected epileptics.

5. Sleep. Sleep as a provocative method is of most use in the diagnosis of temporal lobe epilepsy. Such patients may show only a non-specific abnormal EEG in the waking state, but during sleep, focal epileptic discharges may emerge on the EEG. Barbiturate-induced sleep is therefore often used in the investigation of epilepsy, especially the temporal lobe type. The drug may be given orally or intravenously.

Comment on the use of the **EEG in epilepsy**

Epilepsy is generally diagnosed clinically, but the EEG may be useful in confirming the type of epilepsy and indicating the origin of the abnormal discharge. A single routine EEG record is likely to be abnormal in approximately 60 per cent of cases of epilepsy; this proportion increases markedly if repeated EEG recordings are made and if provocation techniques such as hyperventilation and photic stimulation are employed. Epileptics who are subject to both major and minor fits are likely to have an 'epileptic' EEG.

The commoner types of abnormalities are spikes, slow-waves, and spike and wave discharges, and tend to be of higher voltage than the normal background activity on the EEG.

1. Subcortical (centrencephalic) epilepsy. The neuronal discharge responsible for this form of epilepsy is thought to originate in the upper brain stem or in the thalamic-reticular system, e.g. petit mal. This type of so-called minor fit is associated with a 3 cycles per second spike and wave discharge which is generalised and occurs bilaterally. These discharges are of a much higher amplitude than the background EEG and are readily induced in those subject to petit mal by hyperventilation.

2. Myoclonic epilepsy. These attacks are associated with the appearance of myoclonic jerkings and the EEG often resembles the spike and wave phenomena of petit mal, but there is not the same regularity and the spikes are frequently multiple. This EEG phenomenon is often referred to as 'polyspikes and waves'. These abnormalities are readily induced by sleep or by flickering light.

3. Cortical epilepsy. A disturbance in an area of the cerebral cortex may well provide an epileptogenic lesion and the consequent EEG abnormality comprises either spike, sharp waves or slow waves, or a combination of these. It may not be evident on the original EEG record, especially if the process arises from one or both temporal lobes, but a sleep record or the use of sphenoidal electrodes may augment the appearance of a temporal lobe EEG abnormality. The placement of sphenoidal leads allows electrodes to come into closer proximity to the temporal lobes of the brain than is possible with ordinary scalp electrodes. Temporal lobe epilepsy (sometimes called psychomotor epilepsy) is frequently associated with an EEG which shows evidence of centrencephalic discharge as well as focal cortical discharge, therefore bilateral discharges in the theta range may be seen in association with psychomotor attacks and later the EEG gives way to focal slow activity reflected from the affected temporal lobe. Clinically, patients with temporal lobe epilepsy may be subject to both psychomotor attacks and to attacks of grand mal.

4. Hypsarrhythmia. This occurs in infants and is associated with abnormal epileptic discharges arising in both the cerebral cortex and subcortical structures. The EEG usually shows both spikes and large slow waves and may be of help in diagnosis and in monitoring the effects of treatment with ACTH.

Chronic epileptics with permanent brain damage have a reduced or absent alpha rhythm with widespread theta activity.

Commonly used drugs which alter the EEG considerably are barbiturates which produce fast activity and chlordiazepoxide (Librium) and similar compounds which tend to abolish epileptic discharges.

Describe the EEG changes in **delirium and confusional states**

These conditions may be caused by general systemic disturbances as well as local brain conditions and the EEG abnormality tends to increase with the degree of interference with the level of consciousness. In confusion the EEG becomes slower and shows theta activity, but in delirium or coma the slow activity progresses to a dominant delta rhythm. In deeper coma, when the patient is completely unresponsive, the amplitude of the EEG diminishes and in the terminal stages the EEG becomes flat and featureless. The EEG may be used to assess clinical progress, e.g. during the treatment of uraemia, hepatic coma, severe anaemia and myxoedema.

Comment on the **EEG in dementia**

In senility the frequency of the alpha rhythm tends to become reduced and the amount of faster activity tends to increase. In senile dementia the commonest abnormality is a continuation and accentuation of the features of a senile EEG with resulting slowing of the alpha rhythm. In addition, slow activity, initially theta and often delta activity, becomes manifest. The amplitude of the slow activity is much lower than that seen in acute confusional states and deliria, an important point in differential diagnosis. In arterio-sclerotic dementia the EEG abnormalities may be similar to, though more severe than those occurring in senile dementia, but they may also be absent. In Alzheimer's disease the EEG is almost always abnormal and in the earlier stages is characterised by a reduction in and slowing of the alpha activity with some flattening of the record. Later, slow activity, initially in the theta range but progressing to the delta range, may become evident. In Huntington's chorea the EEG is often abnormal, the alpha rhythm is reduced and the record may be flat. In other forms of pre-senile dementia, e.g. Pick's disease and simple pre-senile dementia, the EEG changes are very variable and the records may be either normal or show a non-specific slow activity.

Comment on the EEG changes in **neuroses and personality disorders**

The majority of individuals in these categories have normal EEGs. Some neurotics may show a reduction in amplitude, or complete disappearance of alpha rhythm with a generalised reduction in amplitude producing a flat record. Fast activity is frequently associated with these changes. Such records are referred to as 'tense' and muscle artefact may be superimposed on the EEG. Psychopaths frequently show immature EEG records, i.e. a considerable amount of theta activity is seen bilaterally in the temporal regions. The incidence of EEG abnormalities in criminals is high, the most frequent abnormality being an immature record.

Describe the **EEG in schizophrenia**

The incidence of EEG abnormalities will vary as much as the clinical picture. At least 50 per cent of schizophrenics have a normal EEG and many abnormalities that occur are entirely non-specific and may be in the nature of (1) epileptiform discharges, (2) low-voltage fast records (tense type of record), and (3) immature records with bilateral temporal theta activity.

Comment on the **EEG in manic-depressive psychosis**

Most of these patients have a normal EEG but it is sometimes possible to see a shift in alpha rhythm to fast frequencies during mania, with slowing during the depressive periods.

Describe the effects on the EEG of major and minor tranquillisers and antidepressant drugs

Chlorpromazine produces activation of the EEG and will often precipitate epileptic discharges in the EEG in vulnerable patients, especially epileptics. Fits have occasionally been reported in non-epileptic patients who have been taking the drug as part of their psychiatric treatment. Amitriptyline (Tryptizol) is an anti-depressant drug which is chemically related to chlorpromazine. Like the latter, it has the ability to evoke epileptiform discharges in the EEG of epileptic patients, thus both chlorpromazine and amitriptyline have been used as activating agents in the investigation of epilepsy. Diazepam (Valium) and other drugs of the benzdiazepine group produce fast activity in the EEG and mask epileptic discharges. They may therefore produce a normal record in an epileptic patient, so they should be stopped for at least a week before an EEG is performed.

Describe the effects of electroconvulsive therapy (ECT) on the EEG

After the first one or two treatments the slow activity in the theta and delta bands produced by the ECT is temporary. The slow activity becomes more persistent as more treatment is administered, and especially if the intervals between treatment are short. After completion of the course of ECT the EEG does not return to normality for four to five weeks.

Briefly describe evoked potentials and comment on possible clinical applications

When a stimulus, whether auditory or visual, is introduced during an EEG recording, the resulting evoked potentials are of various types. A general response is provoked, but it is quite non-specific. It may affect the alpha rhythm or produce some transient discharge of uneven amplitude. The specific response to the sensory stimulus occurs after a precise interval and is most prominent over the area of the cortex related to the type of the sensation and the relevant side of the body which has been stimulated. It is this specific response that is referred to as an 'evoked potential'. Various techniques are now available, e.g. average response computers, to record evoked potentials in the EEGs of patients.

The manifestation of evoked potentials is influenced not only by sensory stimulation but also by such factors as fatigue, drowsiness and habituation.

Evoked potentials are of three main types:

(a) Visually evoked. Abnormal responses are seen in asymmetrical lesions of the brain, e.g. tumour; the presence of a hemianopic visual field defect enhances the likelihood of obtaining this type of evoked potential.

(b) Auditory evoked. Auditory stimulation can be of help in detecting hearing disability in children, including brain-damaged and handicapped. Non-specific potentials arising in the brain or in the muscles of the neck and scalp are often evoked.

(c) Somatosensory evoked. Stimulation, either mechanical or electrical, is applied to peripheral nerves in the fingers, toes, arms or legs. This may help in demonstrating the site of a lesion involving the sensory pathways. An example of the use of this technique in the diagnosis of hysterical hemianaesthesia has been reported.

SECTION 5

GENETICS

*List and define **terms in common use** in genetics*

Segregation is the natural division into two classes by a single hereditary character.

Chromosomes are parallel strands or filaments of a material which can be stained by aniline dyes and are contained in the cell nucleus. They are said to consist of desoxyribose-nucleic acid or DNA and grow like crystals, and in humans each individual carries in his cells two complete sets, one from each parent; these are called *homologous* pairs. The number of pairs varies in different animals and in humans this was accepted as 24 pairs, but with improved techniques only 23 pairs (46 chromosomes) can be identified. They are seen in cells from rapidly growing tissues such as bone marrow or the embryo and in cultured cells. This chromosome apparatus acts as a storehouse of information for the organism and this information is located· in a number of *loci* in the chromosome.

Genes are segments of DNA consisting of large numbers of nucleotides and replication may be achieved by separation of complementary nucleotide chains with the formation of new daughter chains. At one time it was thought that one gene unit occupied one locus on the chromosome, but it is realised that numerous genes can be located in these stations and each gene itself may be a complex of genes.

Homozygous is the term used for a person or animal who carries an identical pair of single genes derived from each parent and under environmental conditions will exhibit the characteristic associated with that gene.

Heterozygous is when the person receives the gene from only one parent and at the corresponding locus of the chromosome there is a different gene from the other parent.

Alleles are the family of elements which are always found at the same locus, the adjective being *allelic*.

77

Dominant is applied to the genes of a heterozygous pair which produce the trait in the offspring. It is frequently preceded by the name 'mendelian' after its originator, Gregor Mendel.

Recessive is applied to the gene of a heterozygous pair which does not express itself in the offspring.

Phenotype is the visible expression of characters in a group of individuals whose heredity is different. A recessive trait should be homozygous before it can be expressed in the phenotype.

Genotype is the fundamental gene formula of an individual. It need not present in the phenotype as in heterozygosity when the gene is carried by the individual but is not expressed by him.

Karyotype is the term used to describe the chromosome picture and is applied to a systematised array of the chromosomes of a single cell prepared by drawing or photography.

Mutation is that variability in the gene structure which is either spontaneous or induced (e.g. by irradiation). There are two kinds recognised:

1. Those which consist of rearrangement, breakage and junction of chromosomes.

2. Those which affect single loci by producing new allelic genes or *point mutations*.

Mutation can account for the spontaneous emergence in several generations of a dominant characteristic which is biologically unfavourable and its subsequent disappearance. Examples are achondroplasia, tuberous sclerosis and retinoblastoma.

Autosomes are those 22 pairs of chromosomes other than the pair carrying the sexual characters which are two X-chromosomes in the female and XY-chromosomes in the male. Distribution of autosomal genes (dominant or recessive) is usually equal between the sexes.

Sex linkage occurs when traits are caused by genes located on that pair of chromosomes which determines sex. It is almost exclusively concerned with the X-chromosome though it should be theoretically possible for gene interchange to occur between the X- and Y-chromosomes. Those genes on the Y-chromosome would determine those characters transmitted exclusively from affected father to sons. Classical examples of sex linkage are colour blindness and haemophilia, and as one sex (usually the female) carries the gene as a recessive and is unaffected, propagation of the condition demands that the gene is present in both partners and is therefore more likely to occur in consanguineous marriages.

Sex may influence autosomal hereditary characters without sex linkage. This is seen in baldness where the endocrine structure of the female protects her from the condition.

Coupling and repulsion. In lower organisms it has been shown that if genes for two traits are close together on the chromosome, they are likely to appear together in the pedigree and if they are far apart they rarely appear together. In man, the search for coupling and repulsion has not been fruitful, largely because of the small size of families and random mating.

Modifier genes are those subsidiary genes which cause quantitative changes in the expression of a major gene which normally bred true (mutation).

Penetrance is that capacity for the gene to express itself, and this can be influenced by a variety of factors which usually operate by reducing penetrance, and in genetic arguments in psychiatry this phenomenon is freely produced to explain the lack of consistency of expression of a gene which is alleged to be homozygous.

Other explanations are incomplete dominance and recessiveness and that the phenotypic expression of a gene is not a fixed entity, but that it merely sets in train a series of events which can be modified by environmental factors as well as by other genes.

How are **genetic factors defined** *in a human population?*

1. *Family histories.* A pitfall in such studies is that one must not assume that because parents have a similar disease to their offspring that this is genetically determined; for example, syphilis may be communicated from parent to child, but we know that this is not a genetic transmission but the transfer of an infection. The *correlation co-efficient* has been exploited in order to define hereditary traits; one approximating to unity would indicate a strong resemblance in the trait in other members of the family and one approximating to zero would indicate practically no resemblance. This form of factor analysis has been too readily accepted as evidence of a genetic factor but statistical validation

may be remote from clinical experience and would suggest that some of the premises of these statistics were false.

2. *Census.* Some circumscribed communities may yield valuable information by this method, but it can be used only when the data is of an unequivocal nature and diagnostic criteria are not in doubt. These reservations almost exclude it in psychiatric studies and apart from some rare biochemical abnormalities which are easily detected such as phenylketonuria, it is not reliable.

3. *Twin studies.* In European communities, twins occur about once in every 88 confinements, but as a number do not survive because of their high infant mortality, the chances of an adult having a twin, instead of being 1 in 44, is 1 in 60. The ratio of identical to fraternal twins is $1 : 2\frac{1}{2}$, suggesting that the incidence of identical twinning is about 1 in 300 confinements. Identical twins are called *monozygotic*, while fraternal twins are called *dizygotic*. Because identical twins may have the same trait does not mean that the trait is hereditary, and this has been exposed by the following example:

If a student of heredity should hail from another planet and be required to use the twin method to find out whether or not people's clothes were a direct consequence of heredity he would find that identical twins were often dressed alike. He would confidently conclude that the choice of clothes was almost an exclusively hereditary trait and might even suppose them to be a part of the natural skin of the human animal by the exercise of superficial reasoning.

4. *Morbidity-risk data.* This is based largely on statistical expertise and the knowledge of a variety of procedures to define the expectancy rates of certain traits. For genetic purposes a common condition is one with an incidence of 1 in 1000 and common genes are liable to modification by 'modifier genes' or by environment. If a single gene is responsible for the condition and the exact mode of transmission is known it should be possible to make a valid prediction, but even then only in terms of probability. Absolute certainty does not exist and a wrong prediction is for the unfortunate parent a 100 per cent error. Even with an established recessive trait the probability of a subsequent child being

affected where one already exists is 1 in 4. In the common mental disorders there is no real point in trying to predict; we just do not know.

What is the basis of **chromosome studies** in genetics?

A colchicine preparation of chromosomes shows them to be nearly split into chromatids, adherent at the centromere. The limbs of the chromatids bend away from the centromere, so that if this is central (metacentric) the structure is X-shaped, and if near the end (acrocentric) it is V-shaped. Each structure is a partly split chromosome and the other member of the chromosome pair is elsewhere in the preparation. The centromere does not stain with the usual stain and therefore presents as a gap. As each chromosome pair has identical length and division of arms, this permits identification.

Describe the **clinical syndromes** associated with chromosomal abnormalities

1. *Trisomy-21* (Down's syndrome). An extra chromosome 21 is generally associated with this condition while a few cases of Down's syndrome have the normal 46 chromosomes, but these are the 'translocation' cases in which the bulk of the extra 21 is still present but attached to another chromosome.

2. *Trisomy-X* (XXX syndrome). This is found in about 1 per cent of female subnormals who may be fertile with normal offspring and is diagnosed mainly by buccal smear which shows the duplicated sex-chromatin bodies in the nuclei. Cases with four or more X-chromosomes occur, but three are by far the commonest.

3. *Trisomy-XY* (XXY Klinefelter's syndrome). This is found in males who in addition to having small testicles and being infertile may exhibit eunuchoidism, gynaecomastia and mental defect. The presence of sex-chromatin in the buccal smear is diagnostic and the condition accounts for over 1 per cent of all male defectives and for 3 per cent of men who are infertile.

4. *Monosomy-X* (XO Turner's syndrome). This is found in females who are usually dwarfed with gonadal hypoplasia, webbed neck, irregular ears and hairline, cubito valgus, shield-shaped

chest with wide-spaced nipples, cardiovascular defects (coarctation) and generally average intelligence.

5. *XYY Phenomenon.* This has been found in an unusually high proportion of aggressive and criminal males detained in special security institutions for the mentally abnormal and subnormal, most of whom were over 6 ft. tall. The full significance of this finding has yet to be determined.

6. *Other abnormalities.* These are being increasingly recognised and trisomics have been described for other pairs. In the main they are found in mentally defective children with multiple congenital defects and multiple trisomics like a Down-Klinefelter combination occur.

What is meant by **chromosomal mosaicism?**

This denotes the presence in one individual of cells which differ in their complement of chromosomes.

What is meant by a **translocation?**

This is an exchange of material between two chromosomes of different pairs (exchange with the other member of the same pair is a normal part of meiosis). This exchange does not have an immediate effect, but as the chromosomes affected are now different from their original partners they cannot pair off properly during meiosis and as a result there are irregularities in the offspring. For example, a translocation may exist which results in the bulk of one 21 chromosome being attached to a larger one. This in itself does not matter and it may continue for several generations, but it affects meiosis so that occasional members of the family acquire an extra dose of 21 and so present Down's syndrome and provide a familial example of the condition. Familial cases of Down's syndrome form the only example of chromosomal anomaly which has to date been recognised as transmissible. All other anomalies cease with the appearance of the case.

SECTION 6

DEFINITIONS

Disturbances of motor behaviour

Negativism is characterised by opposition and resistance to what is suggested. It may be expressed in such forms as mute speech, or in the refusal of food, or behaving in a manner which is directly opposed to what is called for in a particular situation. This form of behaviour may be seen in schizophrenic or hysterical states.

Automatic behaviour (automatic obedience) implies that the patient carries out requests and suggestions automatically. It may manifest itself in a form of behaviour or in repetitive speech (*echolalia*), or by the imitation of movements made by the observer or others (*echopraxia*). These features are seen in catatonic schizophrenia. *Stereotypy* is a repetition of an action or movement and is seen in chronic schizophrenic states. *Mannerisms* are seen in normal people and are not so persistent and monotonous as stereotyped behaviour; they tend to be exaggerated when the subject is under stress. *Compulsions* are morbid and often irresistible urges to perform an apparently unreasonable act; they are frequently seen in children, e.g. touching lamp-posts or not walking on cracks on a pavement. Compulsive acts may assume ritualistic proportions, especially in obsessive compulsive neurosis where the compulsive behaviour is strongly linked to the obsessional thinking. Common compulsions include hand-washing and touching objects several times. *Perseveration* implies the continuation or repetition of a response which is entirely appropriate to the first of two stimuli but is inappropriate to the second one, though it is provoked by it. This leads to abnormally persistent repetition of either speech or behaviour. Perseveration occurs in organic disorders and in schizophrenia.

Psychosis. This term refers to a major mental disorder which is characterised either by deterioration of the personality or by a loss of contact with reality. Psychiatric symptoms such as hallucinations and delusions are often referred to as psychotic features since they occur exclusively in the psychoses. In the neuroses, on the other hand, although disabling symptoms may occur, there is no personality deterioration or impairment of reality testing and no gross impairment of thought processes. It is often said that the neurotic has insight whereas the psychotic has not. There are many exceptions however to this 'rule'.

Disorders of thinking

Flight of ideas means a rapidity in the creation of associations between ideas with a resultant digression from one idea to another. This quickening of the thought processes occurs especially in mania and in hypomania. The term *'clang association'* implies the following of an idea of thought with another which is similar in sound but not in significance. *Retardation* of thought is the opposite of flight of ideas and infers that the flow of thought is abnormally slow. Retardation of thought and of motor activity is seen in psychotic depression and in schizophrenia. *Perseveration* (see above).

Circumstantiality. This is seen where the subject cannot distinguish between essential and non-essential detail; rather tedious digressions are consequently produced. This form of thought, when given verbal expression, is found mainly in organic brain disease and in subnormals. *Over-valued ideas*: the patient, usually a paranoid personality or someone suffering from a paranoid psychosis, attaches great importance to a particular idea which has some special meaning for him, and anything which conflicts with it is not recognised or is denied. The over-valued idea will obviously influence the patient's behaviour to a large extent. *Delusion* is a false, irrational belief which is held with great conviction by the individual, cannot be corrected by logic, reason or suggestion and is not held by others of similar class or culture. Commonly occurring delusions include (*a*) grandiose delusion, (*b*) delusions of persecution (these two types are often referred to as paranoid delusions), (*c*) delusions of guilt and sin, (*d*) nihilistic delusions, (*e*) hypochondriacal delusions. *Ideas of reference:* remarks or behaviour on the part of other people are interpreted by the subject as being referred to him in some significant way. They may attain delusional proportions and are seen in psychotic depression and in paranoid psychoses, e.g.

paranoid schizophrenia. *Obsessional ideas* are thoughts which persistently enter the patient's consciousness against his wish. They usually have a strong emotional component and motivation.

Disturbances of perception

Illusions are distorted perceptions and usually involve visual or auditory stimuli. They may be seen by the mentally normal, in the dark, in the presence of urgent physiological drives or during emotional stress. Illusions occurring pathologically are seen mostly in organic disorders with clouding of consciousness, e.g. delirium.

Hallucinations are false perceptions which occur without the sensory stimuli which characterise illusions. They may be seen in a normal person falling asleep (hypnagogic hallucinations) or in a waking state (hypnopompic hallucinations). A psychosis of any type may be associated with hallucinatory experiences and the commoner hallucinations may involve the various sensory media e.g. auditory, visual, olfactory, tactile and kinaesthetic.

Depersonalisation (see below) is a common symptom which occurs in a variety of psychiatric disorders as well as in healthy people. In some instances it seems to be related to a disturbed perception of self and/or the environment. Thus it is common in LSD intoxication and temporal lobe epilepsy. In these and other states associated with organic brain damage, clouding of consciousness facilitates its occurrence.

Disturbances of affect

Inadequate affect, often referred to as blunting of affect or emotional dulling, usually associated with a general lack of interest and drive and often with personality deterioration, is seen mainly in chronic schizophrenia and in diffuse brain damage. *Incongruity of affect* implies an inappropriateness of emotion or display with incongruous giggling or laughing out of context. This disturbance is seen especially in schizophrenia. *Derealisation* is a common symptom complex in affective disorders, being most frequent in depression and anxiety states. It must be emphasised, however, that it can also occur in normal people, often as a transient feeling. It is seen also in hysterical and obsessional neuroses, schizophrenia and organic mental disorders.

Disturbances of consciousness

Confusion refers to clouding of consciousness with an implied disturbance of awareness. The patient's orientation is disturbed and his general grasp and attention are impaired. It occurs in organic diseases of the brain or other systems. The associated affect is either perplexity or anxiety. *Delirium* is an example of a confusional state (often referred to in the U.S.A. as the acute brain syndrome); hallucinations are present and the patient is markedly agitated and restless. In *stupor* the patient gives every appearance of being asleep but he is in fact unrousable, though he may open his eyes and respond to vigorous stimulation. It occurs in schizophrenic catatonic stupor and in psychotic depression. It may also be caused by disease of the upper brain stem or brain compression, when it is often referred to as akinetic mutism, or it may be associated with drug intoxication. *Depersonalisation* is frequently complained of in states of impaired consciousness, whether due to brain disease, epilepsy or drugs. It has also been reported in subjects undergoing sensory deprivation.

Memory disorders

Amnesia means loss of memory and may be caused by psychological factors, when it is referred to as hysterical amnesia. More commonly it occurs in association with brain disease. *Paramnesia* means falsification of memory or distortions of memory. This is very close to dysmnesia (see below).

Dysmnesia, or the dysmnesic syndrome, or Korsakoff's state. This is associated with poor recent memory and the production of distorted memories (confabulation). The Korsakoff state can be produced by head injury or chronic alcoholism, and is less commonly seen on the basis of cerebral arteriosclerosis, intracranial tumour or following anoxia, e.g. by carbon monoxide poisoning. *Déjà vu*: this is the feeling that something has been experienced before and occurs normally; it also occurs pathologically when it is persistent and causes the patient discomfort. It is often referred to as an illusion of memory and may occur on the basis of a lesion of one or both temporal lobes, consequently it may be seen as part of the aura in temporal lobe epilepsy.

Other 'organic' terms

Aphasia means absence of speech, but the relevant term is usually dysphasia which implies some abnormality of speech. Aphasia or dysphasia may be motor or expressive, or receptive. The latter signifies an inability to appreciate the significance of words whether spoken or written as symbols. *Nominal aphasia*, which used to be referred to as *amnestic aphasia*, produces an inability to identify people or objects by their proper names although the patient is aware of their significance. *Apraxia* is the inability to execute a voluntary movement where there is no impairment of motor or sensory pathways concerned in the control of that movement. It is usually bilateral and sometimes involves the ability to dress or undress (*dressing apraxia*), or to construct models from blocks (*constructional apraxia*). Parietal lobe lesions and dementia are the commonly associated clinical states. *Agnosia* means an impairment of recognition in the visual, auditory or tactile modalities although the primary sensory pathway concerned is intact, e.g. visual agnosia is the inability to recognise seen objects by a patient, whose vision is undisturbed. Lesions are of the appropriate association areas of the cerebral cortex, i.e. visual, auditory or sensory, though the syndrome is often seen in cases of diffuse brain damage, e.g. dementia.

D

SECTION 7

ORGANIC PSYCHIATRY

What is meant by **organic psychiatry?**

At its most general interpretation, all physical illness has its mental accompaniment, if only in the personality of the patient. In addition, many diseases have specific mental features which form an essential part of the clinical picture and which may, because of behaviour disturbances, require treatment in a hospital where such behaviour can be properly evaluated and controlled. This requires the attention either of a psychiatric hospital or of a psychiatric department of a general hospital.

Examples of these diseases are cerebral diseases, such as tumours, degenerative changes, vascular disease and trauma, where the condition may present initially with psychiatric symptoms, like severe depression. In addition there are general medical problems occurring in the psychiatric hospital, for the mentally ill usually have more than their fair share of physical illness. Many theories have been elaborated to explain all mental illness in terms of organic changes while others have claimed that psychiatric problems can in themselves induce an organic change, this aspect being considered one of the features of the psychosomatic disorders which in some respects differ from organic psychiatry.

Briefly then, organic psychiatry is the study of those organic diseases which are commonly associated with psychiatric symptomatology.

Classify the **organic brain syndromes**

These include all cerebral pathology which may lead to mental changes, such as infection, tumour and other space-occupying lesions, vascular abnormalities, trauma, degenerative changes, toxic reactions and encephalopathic states based on biochemical disturbances. They are usually described as *acute* or *chronic* with an intermediate form, *sub-acute*.

88

Acute reaction

Although some authorities have limited this definition to the reversible process, this is unsatisfactory for there are chronic conditions such as pellagra and dementia paralytica which are in fact reversible. The label should therefore be reserved for conditions of acute onset, whether reversible or not. If recovery does not take place, then, as in other medical conditions, it can be said to become chronic.

The clinical picture is that of clouding of consciousness which can range from mild confusion to delirium and coma. Memory may be impaired with lack of concentration and at times distractibility, and in some instances a true dysmnesic syndrome.

Chronic reaction

Though this has been defined by some as an irreversible process, there are objections to this as has been stated under *acute reaction*. Dementia in all its grades is a dominant feature and has been classified under the following headings:

1. A difficulty in retention (the amnesic syndrome).
2. Disturbance of attention, and more particularly, difficulty in focusing attention.
3. Lack of spontaneity, though occasionally there is an excess of spontaneity.
4. Poverty of ideas.
5. Forced responsiveness to stimuli; or perhaps an extreme selectiveness for stimuli.
6. Some degree of disturbed consciousness.
7. Undue tidiness; or on the other hand, slovenliness.
8. Affective disorders.
9. Proclivity to various catastrophic reactions.

Though intellectual defect is usually regarded as the most significant feature of these chronic organic brain syndromes, this may not necessarily be so. Just as in mental deficiency it has long been recognised that intellectual defect is a poor index, social behaviour being far more important, so with dementia. Social, emotional and behavioural deficits are frequently of greater importance. A patient may have lost very little in intellectual functioning, but because of disturbing behaviour, depraved social habits or emotional immaturity, his work and home may reject him. One should consider dementia in a 'global' sense and then one may be able to identify the dementia 'differentials'.

What is **Goldstein's contribution** *to the understanding of the organic cerebral reaction?*

Goldstein, who made an intensive study in soldiers with head injuries during the First World War, has based his conclusions on three methodological postulates.

1. All the phenomena presented by the patient should be considered without giving preference in description to any one, i.e. no symptom is greater or lesser in importance than another.

2. There must be accurate description of the observable phenomena, and not merely a description of their effects, for the effects may not be expressive of the underlying function and in some instances give unreliable information. The 'plus or minus method' of recording can be erroneous, for the result may be achieved by a roundabout way which unless carefully analysed is ignored in the final reading.

3. No phenomenon should be considered without reference to the organism concerned, and to the situation in which it appears.

In addition to these postulates, he has enunciated the following laws:

1. A single performance field will never drop out *alone* for invariably *all* performance fields are affected although the degree to which the individual field is involved varies.

2. A single performance field will never drop out *completely*. Some individual performances are always preserved.

3. Although a patient may present different symptoms in different fields, these symptoms are expressions of the same basic disturbance.

4. The basic disturbance can be regarded as a change of behaviour or as an impairment of brain function and the behaviour change is usually a failure to handle the *abstract* and a retention of the capacity to manipulate *concrete* situations. This principle pervades a variety of responses such as action, perception, thinking and volition. He calls this *disturbance of categorical behaviour.*

Disruption of function first attacks the most highly organised and later the more basic functions are impaired. Consequent on this, there is a gradual loss of the faculties which are most characteristic of the individual till he is left with those of the gross dement. The highest forms he calls 'ordered' and the others he calls 'disordered or catastrophic'. In the 'ordered', responses appear constant, correct and adequate for the respective organism as well as to the respective circumstances. This is not synonymous with normal behaviour. 'Catastrophic' reactions are inadequate, disordered, inconstant and inconsistent and the patient exhibits anxiety.

The patient's conduct may exhibit the following:

1. Tendency to orderliness.
2. Avoidance of 'emptiness'. The patient may exhibit this by rarely using the middle of a sheet of paper to write on, but will write at the top edge and crowd the writing very closely.
3. Relative maintenance of ordered behaviour by shrinkage of the environment in proportion to the defect.
4. Tendency to optimal performance.

What is meant by **perseveration**?

This is a feature found in a variety of organic states. In the clinical sense, perseveration implies the continuation or repetition of a purposeful response which is entirely appropriate to the first of two stimuli but is inappropriate to the second one, though it is provoked by it. The condition is also found in schizophrenic patients and it may be difficult to distinguish the organic from the functional, but fortunately other features in both diseases are usually available to help in the differential diagnosis.

Describe the clinical features of **dementia paralytica** (*general paralysis of the insane*)

This condition used to account for 10 per cent of mental hospital admissions but is now much rarer although in recent years there has been a slight increase in incidence, probably as an aftermath of infections acquired during the Second World War. Venereologists are also concerned about the present tendency for teenagers to acquire venereal infection because of a loosening of moral values and the prevalence of modern contraceptive clinics which are not 'preventative' against venereal disease. Of course, adults are no less at risk.

Pathology

Microscopically. The disease is caused by the organism *Treponema pallidum*, which can be demonstrated in the brain. In addition:

(1) There is cellular infiltration of small vessels and capillaries by plasma cells and lymphocytes, and this is seen particularly in the cortex and corpus striatum. (2) Endarteritis of small cortical vessels. (3) Proliferation of large astrocytes. (4) Intra-adventitial iron deposits. (5) Cell changes in the parenchyma including (*a*) dropping out of nerve cells, (*b*) disturbance of the cytoarchitectonics of the cortex and (*c*) circulatory determined cell changes, such as in the Sommer sector of the *cornu Ammonis*. (6) The lesions are diffuse, but are particularly concentrated in the anterior part of the cortex, decreasing toward the posterior pole with the *cornu Ammonis* being particularly involved. Nerve cell destruction is more marked in the front of the brain.

Physical signs

1. *Speech disorders.* Difficulty in articulation, hesitation and slurring. In the early stages, test phrases such as 'Methodist Episcopal Church' and 'Royal Irish Constabulary' are pronounced incorrectly.

2. *Pupillary changes*, particularly the Argyll Robertson pupil which is found in over 50 per cent of paretics. It is excessively contracted, and though reacting to accommodation does not react to light.

3. *Optic atrophy*, in 50 per cent. This may progress to complete blindness.

4. *Handwriting.* Considerable mis-spelling, omissions and repetitions as well as disorganisation in the formation of the letters. This is partly due to tremor, but is also due to difficulty in arranging things in space.

5. *Tremor* is coarse and is seen in the fingers, lips and tongue, the latter when protruded showing the 'trombone' effect.

6. *Facial appearance* is mask-like with flattening and smoothing of the nasio-labial folds and the faculty of expression and mobility is deficient.

7. *Convulsions.*

8. *Muscular inco-ordination* which is seen in buttoning clothing or in dressing.

9. *Sphincter disturbances* in the terminal stages.

10. *Knee jerks* are usually exaggerated, with ankle clonus and spasticity.

11. *Apoplectic attacks* followed by hemiplegia or more localised lesions.

12. *Aortitis and aneurysm.*

13. *Laboratory findings:*

(*a*) C.S.F. (i) W.R. and Khan test positive in about 100 per cent of untreated cases. (ii) Increase in cells (10 to 50 per ml.). (iii) Increased protein, particularly the globulin fraction. (iv) Paretic lange (colloidal gold) curve, e.g. 5555444322, though it may be tabo-paretic, e.g. 1122345432. If the patient has had an antibiotic such as penicillin, these features may be masked.

(*b*) EEG. Abnormal tracings in the untreated will depend on the severity of the disease, but may be present in 80 per cent. The tracings are not characteristic, but if convulsions have occurred there will probably be evidence to support them. Disturbances will be more likely localised to the frontal region indicating frontal lobe damage. As with the C.S.F., previous therapy tends to mask EEG abnormalities.

Mental symptoms

1. *Memory disturbance.*

2. *Mood* has traditionally been described as grandiose and expansive, with optimism and euphoria, but in fact apathy and dullness are also common and there is a shallow affectivity, the patient being relatively unmoved by events which in the normal would evoke a marked emotional response.

3. *Delusions* are traditionally described as grandiose.

4. *Mental deterioration*, in the early stages, is manifest as tactlessness such as is found after leucotomy and later it extends to impaired judgment with deterioration in behaviour which

extends into the emotional field, the patient being no longer able to make full rapport with those around him and exhibiting conduct lacking the usual aesthetic and moral qualities he once possessed. As dementia progresses it may be associated with violent and destructive outbursts, and with the concomitant march of the general paralysis, the terminal picture is one of complete dementia with complete paralysis. This state is now rarely seen, for antibiotics, if not able to control the dementia, can arrest the paralytic process.

5. *Delirium* is seen in rapidly developing states and may well be associated with an acute meningitic reaction.

A variety of psychiatric syndromes have been described, and these include:

(1) Simple dementing type. (2) Expansive type. (3) Depressed type. (4) Circular type (including manic and depressive features). (5) Schizophrenic type. (6) Lissauer's type. This is usually characterised by unilateral atrophy of either a whole cerebral region or a group of convolutions, and may be associated with aphasia, apraxia and other examples of selective cortical involvement. (7) Tabo-paretic type. (8) Juvenile G.P.I.

Diagnosis

Apart from the W.R. and Khan, the T.P.I. or Treponema immobilisation test is the final court of appeal. This uses a living strain of virulent *T. pallidum* as antigen, thus providing a sensitive and specific index of treponemal disease. It is primarily used to verify the presence of treponema infection in patients whose sera have given positive reactions such as the W.R. but where there is no clinical evidence of treponemal infection.

Treatment

1. *Malaria therapy:*

  (a) *Mosquito.*
  (b) *Malarial blood.*

2. *Penicillin.* This has largely superseded malaria in treatment. Six million units in repository form are usually effective. A further

course is only required if there is deterioration after initial improvement. The Herxheimer reaction is considered to be the major complication, but this is becoming less of a problem and may well be due to more purified forms of penicillin.

3. *Kettering hypertherm.* This is rarely used now and was an artificial means of inducing fever.

4. *Social therapy.* This is needed at all stages of the condition. Even when the patient has not deteriorated the family will need considerable attention, and when the patient has deteriorated the question of disposal will have to be considered.

Prognosis

Untreated G.P.I. is said to be fatal within five years of the onset of symptoms, and as has been said, while penicillin can arrest the infection or prolong life in most cases, it may not restore function completely.

Meningo-vascular neurosyphilis

Psychotic features are dependent on focal lesions which may result in confusion and delirium with occasionally disorientation. In many ways the clinical picture does not differ from that of a stroke.

Describe the clinical features associated with **cerebral vascular disease**

Cerebral arteriosclerosis

This is a very common condition and has been said to account for 21 per cent of first admissions to mental hospitals.

Aetiology

This is complex and various people stress different aspects. Some see the condition as an extension of hypertension, while others blame dietetic factors leading to high levels of cholesterol in the blood with consequent deposition of atheromatous plaques in the vessel walls. Hypertension as an aetiological factor is hotly disputed by some while others are equally antagonistic to hypercholesterolaemia as a factor. The cholesterol theory has given rise to considerable attempts to use diet as a prophylactic measure, but there is no conclusive evidence that it is effective.

Pathology

This is found in both large and small vessels. In the former the atherosclerosis consists of yellowish patches on the internal surface of the artery, though they may be visible from the external surface due to the relatively thin walls of the cerebral blood vessels. In small vessels there is:

(*a*) Diffuse hyperplasia with thickening of the media. (*b*) Hypertrophy of the muscle of the media with increased collagen deposit. (*c*) Hyalinisation of the intima with deposition of hyaline material in the subintimal layer with progression to complete obliteration of the lumen, and the internal elastic lamina is frequently split and fragmented but may also be reduplicated. (*d*) Obliterative cerebral arteriosclerosis.

Symptomatology

As the lesions may be small or large, single or multiple, in areas which are more or less vulnerable and which have their own characteristics, either mental or physical, and where arteriosclerosis may exist without causing symptoms, the clinical features of the disease can be most diverse and the diagnosis very difficult. As a general rule, an organic psychosis occurring after the age of 50 years with negative serology and in the absence of other diseases associated with cerebral involvement, should be regarded as cerebral arteriosclerosis, especially if there is other evidence of this condition.

Prodromal symptoms are easy fatiguability, headaches, giddiness, discomfort in the head and neck, inability to concentrate, drowsiness, character changes and intolerance for alcohol. Neurological features such as temporary loss of power in the extremities, paraesthesiae, transitory aphasia, pupillary inequalities and spastic gait, may also be prodromal and, especially if transitory, may be attributed to spasm of the cerebral arteries, though this phenomenon is still not generally accepted. The presence of supporting evidence such as hypertension, retinal changes of an arteriopathic nature, cardiac (left ventricular) hypertrophy and renal disease will help to establish the diagnosis. A common feature is a confusional episode which may give way to excitement and restlessness indicating cerebral irritation, which is not usually static but can fluctuate with apparently full remission. Frankly psychotic features may present with paranoid ideas, usually of a persecutory nature and auditory hallucinations, the patient changing rapidly from a rational being to one who is mentally disturbed and impervious to reasoning. Those familiar with the patient notice a gradual or sudden falling off in performance which is mainly due to failure to comprehend.

Mental symptoms

1. *Memory defect* is variable but initially is usually limited to forgetting of names, places and recent events. A fluctuating course is the rule and there may be surprising episodes of lucidity.

2. *Personality changes* are varied, but certain features are more common. These include a tendency to eccentricity and a deterioration in personal care, with lack of appreciation of one's surroundings and the ordinary proprieties of social conduct. They may result in sexual aberrations such as indecent exposure, which may be in response to provocative suggestions by little girls in the park, and not due to some compulsion but to a failure to comprehend the real situation. Paranoid features are regarded as an uncovering of the individual's pre-morbid personality.

3. *Emotional responses* are labile but not incongruous. The patient may be easily moved to tears or laughter, but only by situations which would normally evoke a similar response. He is aware of his defects and reacts appropriately, being frequently very distressed by his handicap and occasionally attempting suicide. The mood may be closely linked with the thought content and in paranoid reactions the patient may be very suspicious, hostile or overtly aggressive and occasionally homicidal.

Course and prognosis

The course of the deterioration may be varied in nature as well as in time, and patients may become childish and quarrelsome, elated, hypochondriacal, deluded and hallucinated, but the steady march of a failure in comprehension is common to all and they frequently distress their families by failing to recognise them or by misidentifying, e.g. daughter for a wife. This disorientation may be reinforced by hallucinatory experiences, the patient insisting that a close relative is in the ward and he may disturb the other patients in his search for the source of the auditory hallucination. Death may occur from a cerebral catastrophe, but cardiac, pulmonary and renal complications take their toll.

Treatment

No specific treatment exists, but there are some positive and rational measures which can help. Many of these patients, through dietary indiscretions, are vitamin-depleted and replacement may remove the pellagra-like dementia which occasionally adulterates the clinical picture. Restlessness can be effectively controlled with sedatives like chloral hydrate 1·0 g. while tranquillisers such as chlorpromazine can deal with the acute hallucinatory episodes. Dosage will depend on the severity of the disturbance, but 100 mg. t.d.s. may be necessary in very severe cases. Prolonged administration of bromides could lead to bromism, which may be difficult to recognise in the presence of cerebral arteriosclerosis.

These patients are not able to adjust to frequent changes of location and the family should be encouraged to have the patient stay at home with the one relative rather than move him about to share the burden.

Write a short note on the **psychology of ageing**

The changes in performance with age are:

1. Slowing of sensorimotor activities.
2. Impairment of short-term memory.
3. Difficulty in relating what is perceived to the required action.

All changes with ageing are not disadvantages. An increased ordering of knowledge with a rise in 'information' scores and improvement in vocabulary are commonly found. Neither does ability to learn decline with age to the extent commonly supposed.

What are the **organic senile psychoses?**

These can depend on the underlying pathology. If this be cerebral arteriosclerosis, the symptomatology is similar to that in the younger age-groups; vitamin deficiencies such as nicotinamide produce a pellagra-like state; anoxia produces its periods of confusion as does uraemia, hepatic involvement, drugs, etc.

Discuss the ageing mind

The impairment of memory sets in motion a chain of events which produces the stereotype of the ageing mind: (1) there is increasing difficulty in recognising persons and objects; (2) defective orientation for time and place; (3) illusionary states regarding surroundings and even their own person; (4) sudden amnesic crises may develop and the individual may be found wandering about the street with no knowledge of his name or address; (5) dreams are not separated from the waking state and the patient literally lives in a dream world mixing dreams with reality; (6) disturbances in sleep rhythm further confuse the patient's orientation for time; and (7) as a result of these developments, frank delusions and hallucinations supervene, but these are in a setting of confusion rather than that of clear consciousness found in the functional states.

Affective disturbances

These are commonly grafted on to the senile process, and should they present early the differential diagnosis between a severe depressive illness and early senile dementia can be very difficult. Depressive delusions are similar to those seen in senile depression, with hypochondriasis, poverty and persecution high on the list. Suspicions of being robbed, which are partly based on impaired memory and partly on the unmasked psychotic process, are also common. These suspicions may become frankly paranoid, the patient accusing his life-long partner or his devoted children of trying to rob and to murder him and frequently embarrassing his family by repeating these allegations to complete strangers.

Behaviour disturbances

These may either accompany the initial psychotic features or develop later. Aggression and violent behaviour may supervene. Deterioration in habits with loss of the patient's normal regard for cleanliness and attention to his toilet, may make it impossible for the patient to remain at home. The condition, like dementia paralytica, may on occasions be ushered in with delinquent behaviour such as indecent exposure, pilfering, mouthing obscenities or sexual assaults.

Pathology

Brain shrinkage is common but may not be the cause of the dementia, for normal senile brains are also shrunken with widened sulci. Subdural haematomata are not uncommon, and it is as well to bear this in mind when seeing the patient, for some may respond to surgical treatment.

Microscopically there is a reduction of cortical nerve cells and granulo-vacuolar degeneration. Senile plaques are present and some try to equate the number of senile plaques with the degree of deterioration, but this is still unproven.

What is meant by **presenile dementia?**

Definition

Presenile dementia is a state of intellectual and/or emotional impairment due to organic cerebral change occurring before the age of 65 years. A large variety of disorders are responsible and include space-occupying lesions, cerebrovascular diseases, trauma, infections, poisons of external origin, such as alcohol, barbiturates and carbon monoxide, vitamin deficiencies, such as nicotinic acid, endocrine deficiencies such as thyroid, and degenerative disorders like Huntington's chorea. These will be described under their various headings and the following descriptions apply to the idiopathic presenile dementias of Alzheimer and Pick, or Alzheimer's disease and Pick's disease as they are called.

Alzheimer's disease

Histopathology. There is atrophy of cortical nerve cells and within the cortex are argentophile plaques which are demonstrable by silver-impregnation techniques. The plaques have a mixed granular and fibrillary structure and silver staining shows irregular thickening and disorientation of the nerve cell fibrils which form 'tangles' and 'loops'. Staining of biopsy material shows coarsely granular clumps which stain positively with periodic acid-Schiff technique (PAS) at the site of the argentophile plaques.

Macroscopically the brain is atrophied with widening of the sulci mainly in the frontal and parietal regions though the rest of the cortex may also be involved.

Differential diagnosis of Alzheimer's disease from the other primary presenile dementias such as Pick's disease and Jakob-Creutzfeldt's disease are shown in the following table:

Clinical features	Alzheimer's disease	Non-Alzheimer's disease
Memory loss . . .	Early	Late
EEG changes . . .	Early	Late
Apraxia . . .	Early	Late
Fits	Late	Early
Incontinence . .	Late	Early
Neurological signs . .	Late	Early
Confabulation . . .	Late	Early
Personality changes . .	Late	Early
Psychotic symptoms . .	Late	Early

Pick's disease

This is another primary presenile dementia which is also called circumscribed lobar atrophy, the frontal and temporal poles being most affected. Because of the frontal lobe damage, behavioural and emotional changes are more commonly seen and the clinical features are generally those represented in the table above in the non-Alzheimer group.

Discuss the aetiology, *clinical features and the treatment of* **Huntington's chorea**

The disease was originally described by Huntington in 1872 in the descendants of three men who hailed from Bures in Suffolk and who had emigrated to New England in 1630. It is a degenerative disease of the central nervous system which results in choreiform movements and dementia and is said to be inherited as a pure Mendelian dominant, though instances have been described where there was no evidence of a family history.

Neuropathology

Macroscopically the brain is small, particularly in the frontal regions with marked atrophy of the gyri, and especially of the corpus striatum, which is seen on coronal section. The ventricles are enlarged and the internal capsule is relatively broad. *Microscopically* there is atrophy of the corpus striatum with degeneration and destruction of the ganglion cells, particularly in the posterior part of the putamen, the globus pallidus being intact.

Clinical features

These may vary considerably. It is insidious in onset and may be ushered in either with personality changes or with the choreiform movements or both and usually starts in the 30s or 40s. Early psychiatric features are moodiness, irritability and neglect of home and person. In the later stages, frank psychotic features are evident and they range through delusions of persecution, religiosity, aggression and grandiose behaviour. Dementia is progressive and an intolerance of alcohol may also occur.

The choreiform movements may go unrecognised for some time, for in the early stages it may be merely an involuntary twitch of a digit or a facial grimace which might pass as a mannerism. These may disappear when the patient is aware he is being observed. Hemichorea or bilateral chorea with grimacing, explosive speech and spluttering as well as athetoid movements of the hands are seen. The gait may become ataxic, and occasionally in the gross case there is a peculiar gyrating movement. A rarer presentation is a respiratory form where the patient's breathing becomes affected.

Treatment

The phenothiazines can contribute a measure of relief, the most effective being thiopropazate (Dartalan). Dosage of 30 mg. per day is usually given.

What is meant by **low-pressure hydrocephalus** and how is it diagnosed?

This is a relatively rare condition which presents as presenile dementia and is in some instances amenable to surgical intervention in the form of creating a ventricular shunt. It was diagnosed by pneumo-encephalography but more recently isotope encephalography using RISA (radio-active iodinated human serum albumin) and an E.M.I. brain scan have proved useful. Three patterns of RISA scan are defined:

1. No trace appearing in the cortical subarachnoid space.
2. An intermediate pattern where some appears.
3. Pure cerebral atrophy.

In group 1 dramatic results may be obtained but in group 2 results are disappointing.

The advantages of using RISA and a brain scan over air encephalography are:

1. It gives a more reliable index of patency of the cortico-subarachnoid channels.
2. Ventricular isotype activity always pointed to an obstruction.
3. It is safer to use, for air studies in these patients can be very traumatic.

What are the **psychiatric aspects of head injury?**

The psychiatric aspects of head injury include functional and organic factors and frequently a mixture of both.

They are usually divided into *acute*, which includes concussion, and *chronic*. The vast majority of concussed are uncomplicated. The patient loses consciousness after the injury, and when he regains it he may show nothing more than a post-traumatic amnesia. Some may not even be unconscious, but behave automatically, though purposively and even effectively. Many a footballer has been concussed, but has not lost consciousness and has continued to play and score goals. After the game he has had no memory whatever for the events following the blow on the head. A similar situation has been described in boxers.

The mechanism is still debated, and the idea that it was due to cerebral ischaemia is now discounted.

Punch drunk. This most often affects professional fighters of the slugging type, who are usually poor boxers and who take considerable head punishment, seeking only to land a knockout blow. There is a high correlation between clinical symptoms and EEG patterns, the latter being more grossly disturbed in the less able boxers. Because of the suspect initial mental equipment of people who take up professional boxing the existence of a syndrome has been seriously questioned in terms of its boxing aetiology. The condition is still under active study and it remains to be seen whether it can be directly attributable to boxing or whether other factors play a more important part. Many workers have found great difficulty in excluding a pre-existing brain defect or coincidental disease. At one time abnormalities of the cavum septum pellucidum demonstrated by air encephalography were regarded as specific, but this now is also disputed.

Traumatic coma. This is a frequent result of severe head injury and the psychiatrist's interest is mainly confined to the dysmnesic (Korsakoff) state which may result from it.

Traumatic delirium. This has to be distinguished from other causes of delirium and can be a very difficult task, particularly when alcoholic delirium is being considered. A person who has been in an accident and perhaps concussed may be given some spiritous drink by a benevolent bystander and the doctor will then be confronted by a delirious patient who is smelling of drink. Worse still, an alcoholic in the course of a bout may fall and injure his head and then present with delirium. A thorough physical examination and admission to hospital is essential when faced with such a problem.

Korsakoff's syndrome. This is frequently referred to as the *dysmnesic syndrome* and is a common sequel of head injury. It may present with a classic confabulatory state as seen in the alcoholic Korsakoff. It usually recedes and there is an interesting phase when the disorientation for time, place and person gives way to an 'as if' phenomenon. The patient begins to appreciate his surroundings but still cannot believe he is in hospital. He may say that he knows he is in hospital, but that he feels he is in a factory and that the doctor reminds him of the foreman and so on. This usually gives way to full insight, though some do become chronically handicapped.

Subdural haematoma. This is alleged to be on the increase and is attributed to three factors: (1) the increased number of head injuries; (2) the increasing life expectancy (most patients are aged 40 to 70 years); and (3) increased awareness of the complications.

Post-concussion syndrome. The psychiatric symptoms are inability to concentrate, fatiguability and impairment of memory with anxiety features. Although these can be evidence of early dementia, they may also represent a purely functional disturbance, and evidence of even severe head injury does not mean that the symptoms are organically determined, for many with brain damage completely recover their faculties and there must be a number who hold distinguished office who have at some time sustained a severe head injury, including the loss of brain tissue.

Functional disturbances

Many symptoms have been attributed to organic causes, on the evidence that the patient had such an injury and that such symptoms frequently occur in patients who have had these injuries. That similar symptoms occur in patients who allege they have had a head injury but have not, or who have injured another part of the body, and also in patients with phobic anxiety, is frequently ignored by those with an organic bias. Nor do they explain why most severe head injuries do not develop these sequelae—why footballers can head goal posts and be unconscious for several minutes, resume the game and be fit for work on the Monday; and why steeplechasers can be thrown from their horses, lose consciousness and then remount; nor do they explain why a housewife can sustain many bumps on the head while at home and be relatively symptom-free, but should she knock her head ever so gently while cleaning at an office or while on a bus which brakes suddenly, the post-traumatic or post-concussion syndrome presents in its most florid form.

What **investigations** would be useful in case of head injury?

1. *Electroencephalography*. In the acute stage the EEG may show bursts of high voltage 2 to 3 c./s. waves, while in the chronic stage the voltage is generally low and the frequency is of the region of 2 to 7 c./s. The disturbance is generally proportional to the severity of the injury and the persistence of symptoms. It is not uncommon for the problem to be adulterated by drugs, particularly barbiturates, which can influence the EEG either by producing fast waves, or in severe intoxication, slow waves and occasionally fits.

2. *Radiography*. Pneumoencephalograms are reputed to be abnormal in 80 per cent of patients who have symptoms related to old head injuries. The commonest finding is a generalised enlargement of the ventricles, though this may not necessarily be pathological.

3. *Psychological tests.* Theoretically these should be of great assistance, but in practice they do not offer much help in diagnosis. The patient may score badly due to lack of motivation and this lack may or may not be caused by his organic mental state. Of greatest help is a comprehensive test like the Wechsler Adult Intelligence Scale (WAIS), which because of its variety of sub-tests shows whether there is a general depression of performance, which may be due to functional factors, or whether there are deficiencies in certain operational fields. Should the latter prove to be the case, then organic factors are more likely to be operating.

Projection tests may be of some help, but are unlikely to be conclusive. Creativity is said to be impaired after brain damage, but as there is unlikely to be any pre-traumatic standard by which the deterioration can be measured, it is difficult to draw any conclusions, as most creative artists without any head injury or brain damage would score very differently at different times in a test designed to measure creativity.

Discuss the **personality changes** *in head injury*

This is a most controversial field. Loss of interest, irritability, moodiness, apathy, outbursts of temper, are all quoted as post-traumatic personality changes and it is extremely difficult at times to say whether these are organically or functionally determined. It has been shown that those who had a personality handicap after head injury usually had a pre-traumatic history of poor inter-personal relations. Others have been unable to distinguish between the symptomatology of post-concussion patients and those with a common neurosis. Generally, in personality changes following head injury the brain damage is of secondary importance, and the pre-traumatic personality is of primary importance in determining the nature of those changes. It is generally agreed that in the absence of neurological signs, or an abnormal EEG, there is no personality change which could be directly attributed to the head injury.

Prognosis

The eventual outcome in cases of severe head injury is usually much more favourable than had been predicted.

Treatment

Early rehabilitation is essential. This is particularly important in brain damage, for the patient should be encouraged to perform up to his capacity as soon as he is deemed capable of doing so. If deficit has resulted from the injury, various adaptive responses will have to be learned and the sooner these are acquired the less the permanent handicap will be. Drugs should be used with great discretion, and although barbiturates are considered a useful prophylactic against the development of post-traumatic epilepsy, they have their drawbacks in that they potentiate personality changes and generally slow the patient down; if excessively prescribed they can produce a state akin to dementia, as well as addiction.

Discuss the psychiatric aspects of disseminated or **multiple sclerosis**

A disease which produces discrete lesions in the brain, some subcortical and others in the region of the brain stem and which is liable to sudden exacerbations, is likely on occasions to be responsible for mental changes. The commonest is emotional lability, and though it used to be taught that euphoria is a conspicuous feature, depression may be at least as common, if not as conspicuous. As with other organic cerebral states, the predisposition of the underlying personality will strongly colour the psychiatric picture and paranoid reactions are not uncommon. The emotional lability, with fleeting and at times indefinite neurological signs, used to be responsible for labelling the condition hysteria, but this was before the dawn of dynamic psychiatry with its emphasis on defining an adequate and fully relevant psychopathology, and before the dawn of the Babinski reflex and the more rigid exclusion of the organic.

It is not possible to define a specific personality type, but evidence of progressive intellectual deterioration has been demonstrated. Although dementia as a sequel is recognised, there are many patients of long-standing who do not deteriorate mentally though it would appear that the dementia aspect in general cannot be divorced from the general progress of the disease.

Depression in disseminated sclerosis is usually most difficult to assess because of the emotional lability with tendency to tearfulness which the organic nature of the condition may provoke. It is an even more difficult problem as far as treatment is concerned. It is known that ECT can aggravate the condition and therefore the most effective treatment for depression is denied, and one has to resort to antidepressant drugs. Imipramine hydrochloride is generally effective even in very severe cases.

Describe the psychiatric aspects of **Schilder's disease**

The symptomatology in Schilder's disease will depend largely on the site of the lesion, which is that of a diffuse sclerosis, though there may be some discrete areas of demyelinisation which histologically can resemble disseminated sclerosis. It is usually rapidly progressive and presents with cortical blindness, though optic atrophy and papilloedema have also been reported and the differential diagnosis from a cerebral tumour can prove very difficult, especially as headache, vomiting and vertigo may precede the grosser neurological picture. Mentally, the features may vary tremendously, and diagnoses ranging from hysteria to dementia, by way of schizophrenia, have been made. There is usually impairment of comprehension which deteriorates to confusion and dementia, and mixed psychotic features occur while the patient is still mentally capable of elaborating them. The prognosis is poor, deterioration is rapid and the challenge to the psychiatrist is likely to come in the early phase of the illness, when he may be asked to see a patient presenting with rather ill-defined psychiatric symptoms. A careful physical examination should reveal the organic nature of the condition.

Schilder's disease is generally regarded as a cause of mental defect since it occurs more commonly in children, but adult cases are not unknown.

Discuss the psychiatric aspects of **brain tumour**

The brain is the commonest site of neoplasms which are most likely to present with psychiatric symptoms and frequently these symptoms may be the earliest indication of intracranial disease. Furthermore, the first physical signs of the brain tumour may be precipitated by psychological stress, and this may prove a difficult problem in differential diagnosis. The commoner psychiatric features of brain tumour are:

1. *Dementia*, which may extend from slight impairment of memory to gross cerebral deficit including Korsakoff's psychosis.

2. *Epileptic phenomena*, which may resemble the features of temporal lobe epilepsy.

3. *Hallucinations*, which are rarely auditory but are usually visual, olfactory or tactile.

4. *Mood disturbance*. Depression and mania may be associated with temporal lobe lesions, and depression is a frequent early symptom of an acoustic neuroma.

5. *Disorders of speech*, particularly dysphasia.

The localisation of the brain tumour may be manifest by specific symptoms.

1. *Frontal lobe*. There is frequently a disturbance of the ability to synthesize perceptions and as with other areas of brain deficit there is less capacity for abstract or creative thought. On the other hand, a patient may have extensive frontal lobe damage and lose relatively little faculty. Personality changes are tactlessness, apathy and *Witzelsucht* which is a tendency to make feeble puns and jokes.

2. *Temporal lobe*. This presents all the features of temporal lobe epilepsy, and as it carries much of the responsibility for speech and memory, any such disturbance may indicate a temporal lobe lesion.

3. *Parietal lobe*. Apraxia sometimes deteriorating to difficulties with dressing and feeding and finding one's way around.

The nature of the brain tumour itself may present different psychiatric forms. A rapidly growing one like a glioblastoma may present as an acute mental upset with depression, with confusion and dementia following rapidly. A slowly developing meningioma and astrocytoma, depending on their site, can simulate mental illness, particularly initially when there are no localising signs. Cerebral metastases from bronchial carcinoma may present with mental symptoms and with an associated central neuropathy; there may be dementia.

What are the psychiatric features of **epilepsy**?

These are so wide and varied that they may include an example or distortion of every feeling or movement of which the patient is capable, in an infinite number of variations and combinations. The major features include disturbances of sensory experience and consciousness as well as motor activity, and the range is wide. Epileptic hallucinations are also present and may involve the special sensations of a unitary or complex nature. Paranoid psychoses and fugue states can occur.

What is meant by **hystero-epilepsy?**

This is a borderland diagnosis which is used when it is impossible to distinguish between the hysterical and organic nature of the attack. Some have doubted its clinical validity, whereas others have linked it with temporal lobe epilepsy.

Enumerate the **factors aggravating epilepsy**

1. Hypoglycaemia which either by itself or in a vulnerable person can produce fits. Frequently the blood sugar is not sufficiently low and a constitutional cerebral dysrhythmia must also be postulated.

2. Alkalosis due to excitement with consequent hyperventilation.

3. Hydration which is frequently seen after excessive beer drinking and gives rise to the erroneous assumption that the disturbed behaviour was due to alcohol.

4. Flicker and rhythmic sounds, which may account for some examples of explosive behaviour in trains or on watching a poorly adjusted television set.

Describe the clinical features of **narcolepsy**

This is an invincible need for sleep, usually of short duration at varying intervals, but frequently several times a day and causing the patient to fall down or to lie down in order to avoid falling. The episodic nature of the condition has suggested to some an epileptic basis, but EEG studies do not show the characteristic tracing and in fact the record would pass for normal sleep. It usually occurs in young males and various aetiologies have been postulated including encephalitis, pituitary disorders and psychological factors.

Treatment

This is still dextro-amphetamine sulphate and doses of 50 mg. b.d. may be necessary. The danger of amphetamine addiction which is now widely recognised has led to a re-appraisal, not only of the use of amphetamine in the treatment of narcolepsy but of the nature of the condition itself. The condition is frequently associated with marked depressive features, the hypersomnia acting as a refuge from the depression. More effective antidepressant treatment, such as imipramine, frequently clears the narcolepsy.

What is meant by psychomotor epilepsy?

This refers to epileptic fits which involve disturbances of psychological function and/or behaviour. In 85 per cent of cases there is a lesion of one or both temporal lobes. There is often no loss of consciousness, although some cases are subject to attacks of grand mal in addition.

What is the relationship between endocrine disturbances and mental illness?

Endocrine changes can produce overt physical changes which may influence physique, mental energy and facial appearance, and these may in turn draw the attention and comments of others and cause increasing sensitivity on the part of the patient. Under these circumstances endocrine abnormality contributes to the mental illness via psychological channels rather than physical ones. Examples are Klinefelter's syndrome, Fröhlich's syndrome, gynaecomastia, masculinising tumours in girls, dwarfism and giantism.

There are endocrine diseases which produce mental symptoms directly and these can be best described under the various organs.

The thyroid

Hypofunction (myxoedema) is associated with depression of mood and psychomotor retardation, the mental component frequently deteriorating to a state bordering on dementia. In the advanced state delusions and hallucinations occur, but diagnosis is not necessarily made on the mental symptoms but on the facial appearance and the other evidence of myxoedema. Paranoid features and irritability are common, but these are not specific to the disease. Hypothermia is also found and may be missed unless a low-temperature recording thermometer is used.

Treatment is as for myxoedema with adequate dosage of thyroid, but this replacement must be done slowly otherwise the mental state may be aggravated. In the ordinary case, 30 mg. daily for the first two weeks should suffice, but insensitive patients may have to be given as much as 300 mg. per day as a maintenance dose. There is a risk in giving chlorpromazine for the control of the acute psychotic features as this may aggravate the hypothermic coma.

Hyperthyroidism is not infrequently associated with mental symptoms, but the clinical picture may vary and resemble either acute mania with motor restlessness, while occasionally visual and auditory hallucinations may predominate. Depression and paranoid reactions may also occur, but in general, hyperthyroid patients are excitable and nervous with undue irritability, jumpiness and over-anxiety in some instances. Treatment is for the hyperthyroidism.

Myasthenia gravis is of psychiatric interest in that it may be aggravated by hysterical features, or it may in fact be simulated by hysterical features. A pseudo-diagnosis is usually based on the following evidence:

1. A history not consistent with myasthenia gravis, either in course, distribution of weakness, relation of weakness to motor activity or response to cholinergic agents.

2. Evidence of significant emotional illness.

3. Absence of weakness on physical examination and inconsistencies on muscle testing.

4. All laboratory findings within normal limits.

5. Lack of uniform improvement in strength following neostigmine and Tensilon.

6. Bulb ergographs of normal or hysterical pattern.

7. Normal motor response to repetitive nerve stimulation.

Pituitary

A basophile adenoma may induce Cushing's syndrome, the psychiatric features of which are varied and can range over the whole field of psychotic reactions but most common are depression and irritability. Polydipsia with polyuria is associated with post-pituitary dysfunction but this condition is frequently found in non-organic states, and differential diagnosis can be extremely difficult. In functional polydipsia there is usually other evidence of psychiatric disturbance in that the polydipsia is essentially compulsive drinking and the patient may be of limited intelligence.

Adrenal cortex

If there is excessive activity there may be the development of a Cushing's syndrome with the psychiatric features already described. If the adrenocortical activity is insufficient, Addison's disease develops, and this is frequently associated with depression as well as anergia and loss of interest and may well be mistaken for a functional state. The depression may deteriorate to serious suicidal risk and therefore it is important that the physical condition be not missed, for psychiatric treatment would be inappropriate. Once the insufficiency is controlled the depression may clear dramatically.

Hypoglycaemia. A long history of progressive mental disturbance with periods of amnesia and confusion, which may lead to a diagnosis of hysteria, schizophrenia or organic dementia, is not uncommonly found in patients with an islet cell tumour of the pancreas with over-secretion of insulin. The mental symptoms are so protean that a variety of psychiatric diagnoses may be made. An EEG may yield a record suggestive or even confirmatory of epilepsy, and the diagnosis is usually established on Whipple's triad of (1) neuropsychiatric symptoms after fasting, (2) a concomitant blood-sugar level below 50 mg. per 100 ml. and (3) banishment of symptoms by the administration of glucose.

It may be difficult to distinguish functional hypoglycaemia from that due to an islet-cell tumour of the pancreas, though the latter usually occurs after fasting while the former may occur two to three hours after a meal. Functional hypoglycaemia when it occurs in the presence of phobic anxiety states may right itself when the psychiatric condition has been successfully treated.

What role does **anaemia** play in mental disorder?

Anaemia and consequent anoxic states can be associated with mental disturbance although the mechanism is not clear. In susceptible subjects quite a small drop in haemoglobin can uncover a florid psychotic state usually of a paranoid nature, though depression and fatiguability are also common features.

Discuss the role of **sensory deprivation** *in mental illness*

Certain subjects, particularly elderly people and people with anoxic states, are susceptible to sensory deprivation, particularly light. In a darkened room they may become vividly hallucinated and this may clear when the light is switched on. Even when normal subjects are deprived of light, meaningful sound and tactile experience, a psychotic pattern, usually of a delusional nature, may supervene after some time. Similar sequelae have been demonstrated by the injection of anaesthetics which deprive the individual of all bodily sensations but leave him conscious. The importance of this work in relation to prolonged space travel or other prolonged exposure to abnormal conditions such as underwater exploring, is self-evident.

What are the psychiatric symptoms associated with **bronchial carcinoma?**

In addition to those associated with secondary deposits in the brain there are others which are associated with central neuropathic changes. It is well known that neurological changes are common in bronchial carcinoma and as many as 40 per cent of patients with neurological changes may show mental abnormalities which are manifest as confusion, depression, stupor, dementia or emotional instability.

Discuss the mental symptoms associated with **vitamin deficiencies**

Wernicke's encephalopathy

Thiamine which is essential for the proper metabolism of carbohydrates and fat and for the normal functioning of the nervous system may, when deficient, cause neurological and psychiatric disturbances. The onset is more acute in children, but in adults it can follow an insidious course which may begin as a neurasthenic syndrome, consisting of anorexia, irritability, emotional lability, lack of concentration and preoccupation with visceral sensations. These may be followed by neurological changes, particularly a polyneuropathy which is bilateral and symmetrical, which initially consists of paraesthesia of toes, burning feet, particularly at night, calf muscle tenderness, and eventually loss of vibration sense and of the ankle jerks, the upper limbs later becoming involved.

The more advanced states in which there is ophthalmoplegia is part of the *Wernicke syndrome* and this includes clouding of consciousness, ataxia and even delirium, although the level of consciousness may appear normal and the patient can present a confabulatory state as is found in Korsakoff's psychosis. A variety of pathological conditions may give rise to this condition such as persistent vomiting as in hyperemesis gravidarum, gastric carcinoma, pernicious anaemia and in malnourished prisoners of war. The ocular signs consist of nystagmus in the horizontal and vertical directions as well as paralysis of conjugate gaze. There may be associated cardiac involvement ('beriberi heart') with an enormous enlargement of the heart, oedema and serous effusions, and sudden circulatory collapse. The cerebral lesions consist of a haemorrhagic polioencephalitis with the mammillary bodies being particularly affected. The laboratory findings include a raised fasting blood pyruvic acid level, but it may be induced by the metabolic stress of 100 g. of dextrose or after exercise.

Treatment lies, as for pellagra, in prevention by giving an adequate diet containing yeast, whole grains, meat, eggs, vegetables and reinforcing the bread ration with a complement of thiamine 1·5 to 2·5 mg. per day. A therapeutic dose is 10 to 100 mg. per day, but in an acute Wernicke state 50 to 100 mg. subcutaneously or intravenously twice daily should be given until a therapeutic result is obtained or the urine indicates tissue saturation by the strong smell of thiamine.

Pellagra

Pellagra is said to present with the classical triad of diarrhoea, dermatitis and dementia. The dementia is not necessarily a mental state exhibiting intellectual deficit but may show behaviour disturbance or psychotic and neurotic features. It is still endemic in certain parts of the world where there is a deficiency of the essential food factors, niacin or nicotinic acid, niacinamide or nicotinamide, and the amino acid precursor, tryptophan. Protein containing tryptophan can compensate for a low niacinamide intake, and this explanation is given for the greater protection derived from tryptophan-containing proteins like wheat, eggs and milk, as against corn protein which is deficient in tryptophan. Countries where the inhabitants live on a high maize diet are likely to have endemic pellagra, and in areas where corn is the main cereal, a toxic niacin-neutralising factor in the corn may be responsible. Factors which singly or in combination may give rise to pellagra are:

1. Dietary deficiencies due to poverty, famine, food fads, ignorance, alcoholism and drug addiction.

2. Low intake due to anorexia, vomiting, disease of the alimentary tract or psychiatric illness including dementia.

3. Impaired biosynthesis due to inadequate intake of tryptophan or the bactericidal effects of antibiotics, since the intestinal flora is responsible for processing much of the body's niacin.

4. Malabsorption.

5. Interference with its use because of generalised impaired cellular metabolism.

6. Interference with storage as in cirrhosis of the liver.

7. Increased excretion as in lactation, diabetes and renal disease.

8. Increased requirements as in pregnancy, rapid growth, high metabolic rate, fever and motor excitement.

9. Extensive post-operative use of dextrose infusions without preventive vitamin therapy.

Mental symptoms may present in three ways: (1) A non-specific neurasthenic syndrome in which the patient may complain of fatiguability, headaches, irritability, inability to concentrate and forgetfulness. (2) An organic psychosis with memory impairment, disorientation, confusion and even confabulation may supervene. It may be associated with excitement, depression, mania or delirium, but paranoid reactions are also common. (3) The encephalopathic syndrome is commonest after a period of delirium and consists of clouding of consciousness, cog-wheel rigidities of the extremities, and uncontrollable sucking and grasping reflexes.

Treatment should be mainly preventive to ensure that everybody has an adequate intake of the vitamin, and niacin-enriched bread has proved to be successful. The average requirements for an adult are 5 mg. of niacine per 1000 calories or approximately 10 to 15 mg. per day. When the disease is present, 300 to 1000 mg. of nicotinamide per day should be given in divided doses, depending on the severity of the disease. In the presence of diarrhoea or when the patient will not co-operate with oral therapy, 100 to 250 mg. should be given by subcutaneous injection two to three times per day, while in the encephalopathic state 1000 mg. by mouth and 100 to 250 mg. by injection per day may be necessary. Once the condition is under control, the dose can be reduced to a basic level. Nicotinamide is preferable to nicotinic acid, as in large doses it does not cause vasomotor disturbances. A liberal diet including a generous supply of milk and adequate meat, liver, peas and greens, and which is low in carbohydrates and fats is also recommended.

Pernicious anaemia

The term 'megaloblastic madness' has been coined to describe psychotic states associated with pernicious anaemia which is due to a B_{12} deficiency. The mental symptoms are generally those of depression though paranoid reactions have also been reported, while in patients with organic cerebral involvement confusional features may also occur. The mental changes can precede the clinical picture of pernicious anaemia by up to eight years, so it is important to screen patients for B_{12} deficiency who may present with depression or paranoid features, particularly those who have had a history of gastric surgery as it is not an uncommon sequel of partial gastrectomy.

What are the **psychiatric sequelae of operative surgery?**

Chest surgery. Operations on the heart and lungs are reputed to be followed more frequently by mental disturbances than operations on other organs. It is difficult to ascertain whether this is due to the physical interference which these operations entail, or whether the nature of the operation itself influences the psychological state of the patient. Delirious states have been reported and these have been attributed to the post-operative environment including abnormal sensory experiences. There are several factors involved including electrolyte changes, the general management of the patient, the level of confidence with which he faces the operation, and the post-operative care. Other aspects of these chest surgical problems is the type of anaesthesia as well as the cardiac by-pass with resulting cerebral involvement.

With the rapid increase in transplant surgery particularly renal, as well as the selection of patients for renal dialysis, psychiatric studies on both patients and staff have shown that the latter may be even more vulnerable. They become closely identified with their patients and undergo considerable stress should dialysis be considered no longer suitable or if their patients are not selected for renal transplant. Similar problems are beginning to arise in coronary care units. Other operations which have been associated with mental disturbances are:

Portacaval anastomosis.
Hysterectomy.
Haemorrhoidectomy.
Cataract removal.

Describe the clinical features of **porphyria**

Porphyria, which is an inborn error of metabolism, presents as three types, the congenital, the acute intermittent and the mixed, the first being mainly found in childhood, while the acute intermittent is the one most commonly associated with mental symptoms. The attacks are usually preceded by periods of nervous tension, and acute episodes may masquerade as neurotic or psychotic states. The acute intermittent type, which is usually associated with mental changes, is said to be due to a Mendelian dominant and is familial while the congenital type is said to be transmitted by a Mendelian recessive. The classical triad of abdominal pain, neuropathy and psychotic symptoms is not always present and the diagnosis may have to be made on two or even one of these criteria, with of course a positive urine test, namely the presence of urobilinogen, though this may be negative except in the acute attack.

Biochemistry

The lesion is said to be due to an incomplete synthesis of purines with overproduction of porphyrins and their precursors due to interference with the succinate glycine circle. Neuropathologically there are patchy areas of demyelinisation with at times destruction of axis cylinders.

Porphyria may be aggravated by a variety of drugs which may be given to the patient during an attack. Most of these act on the liver and include barbiturates, alcohol and sulphonamides. It is important, therefore, that barbiturates be not used to produce anaesthesia in these patients, such as prior to the administration of electroplexy.

A rarer form of the condition is *hereditary coproporphyria* which may present as an acute intermittent form, but the coproporphyrins are more in evidence in the faeces than in the urine.

What are the psychiatric associations of **disseminated (systemic) lupus erythematosus?**

These are varied and may be those of anxiety, depression and even schizophrenia, as well as confusional and delirious phases. A number may also show neurological features. As the condition is generally treated with corticoids, some attributed the mental symptoms to this agency, but this is now in doubt as corticoids have been given to patients recovering from the delirious state with no recurrence of the mental symptoms, and a number of patients had developed the condition who had not been having corticoids in its treatment.

What psychotic states are produced by **toxic agents?**

Toxic psychosis is a term which is frequently invoked to describe those states where there is a definable toxic origin. In this category are two large groups: (1) those cases where the patient is so susceptible that even trivial amounts of the agent will precipitate a psychotic illness, and (2) those cases where the agent itself has earned a reputation for precipitating psychosis. In the first instance there is little to be gained in listing all the agents to which susceptible people may react, though individual examples may be useful in explaining some unexpected events. In the second instance, it is helpful to classify those agents that may be responsible for the psychosis.

It is customary to divide the toxic psychosis into two groups: those due to exogenous poisons and those due to endogenous poisons.

E

Exogenous poisons

Bromides

Normally serum bromide is 3 mg. per 100 ml. and symptoms of intoxication rarely occur below a level of 150 mg. per 100 ml., though in senile and arteriosclerotic patients or those with renal damage a lower figure may suffice. The bromide replaces the chloride in the blood, but it is doubtful if this factor alone is responsible for the ensuing mental state. In mild cases there may be irritability, sleep disturbance and slight impairment of comprehension which may progress to restlessness and confusion. Other features are slurring of speech, dehydration with dry skin, ataxia, tremor of tongue, and acne. In the severe cases, the clinical picture is one of delirium with disorientation and altered consciousness. Four psychotic patterns have been described:

1. Simple intoxication.
2. Delirium.
3. Transitory schizophrenia.
4. Hallucinosis.

In the diagnosis, as well as the serum bromide, the EEG may give useful information for the record is sensitive to bromide and intoxication produces a preponderance of slow waves.

Treatment. Stop the bromide, fluid replacement for the dehydration and administer sodium chloride 2 to 4 g. four hourly.

Methyl bromide

This substance is used in refrigeration and in disinfestation. Toxicity is due to the methyl element and not the bromide, for levels as low as 5 mg. bromide per 100 ml. may be toxic. A mild euphoria and lack of concern in handling the material is evident, and this in turn can lead to major over-exposure or chronic recurrent intoxication with irreversible brain damage. Neurological signs consist of coarse tremor, generalised hyperreflexia and inco-ordination of limb movements.

ACTH and cortisone

These have since their inception had psychiatric overtones. As they are both apt to be euphoriants, there is a tendency for some patients to become addicted to them, particularly so in dermatology, asthma and rheumatology clinics. In view of the very large number of patients who have received the drugs and their specific effects on electrolyte balance, surprisingly few cases of overt psychosis occur. Symptoms are varied and include elation, depression and inappropriate affect as well as acute maniacal excitement with hallucinations and delusions.

Lead

This is the commonest of the metallic poisons which are responsible for mental disorder. It is found in children by reason of 'pica' but also affects adults, particularly through its use in industrial processes, where inhalation of toxic compounds may produce psychiatric symptoms of either an acute or chronic nature. The commoner jobs which carry the risk of exposure are lead-paint spraying, lead burning as in the destruction of old batteries or other salvage work, lead enamelling and lead-glass blowing. The symptoms and signs in the milder states are anorexia, abdominal discomfort, constipation, headache and pallor. The more severe features are abdominal cramps, paralysis of the extensor muscles and the 'lead line' round the gums. Blood examination reveals a microcytic anaemia with increased basophilic stippling of the red corpuscles. There is an increased coproporphyrinuria, the blood lead is above 0·1 mg. per 100 ml. and the urinary lead is above 0·1 mg. per litre.

The mental symptoms may be acute or progressive. In the acute stage there is delirium of sudden onset with confusion, tremors, visual hallucinations and delusions, and occasionally convulsions. In the progressive form there is an apathetic state which may masquerade as depression, memory impairment, speech difficulties and confabulation of a Korsakoff type. A milder form presents a neurasthenic picture with irritability, physical weakness and giddiness, but these symptoms may be due to anaemia.

Treatment is firstly prevention and all industries are now alive to the hazard, and rigorous precautions are laid down. Acute poisoning due to ingestion of lead is treated with gastric lavage with magnesium, sodium or aluminium sulphate solutions followed by plain water to remove the lead sulphate that has been produced. Chronic poisoning is treated by deleading with calcium disodium versenate, a chelating agent which forms a stable water soluble compound with metals. In severe lead encephalopathy, it may be necessary to resort to surgical decompression to relieve intracranial pressure.

Mercury

This is not as common a cause of mental disturbance as lead. Psychiatric symptoms are those of a neurasthenic state with irritability and loss of confidence, though it may produce excitement followed by depression. The neurological features, which include a coarse tremor of the orbit, lips, tongue and hands, may be mistaken for a striatal disorder of unknown aetiology, and mercury poisoning should be borne in mind, for it is used in such a variety of trades that it may well provide the answer to an otherwise obscure problem.

Treatment is by dimercaprol (BAL), which is said to be of value in severe cases of nephrosis and in mental disturbance.

Manganese

This is used in many industrial processes and prolonged exposure may produce neurological and psychiatric symptoms. The former are of an extrapyramidal nature due to involvement of the basal ganglia.

Other mental sequelae include outbursts of uncontrollable laughing and crying and general emotional lability of a less dramatic nature. There is, as yet, no specific treatment but removal from exposure may result in an abatement of the mental symptoms, the neurological ones tending to persist.

Discuss the role of **carbon monoxide** in psychiatric illness

This is both a cause and a result of mental disturbance, for it is one of the commoner methods of attempting suicide. It is produced by car exhausts, mine explosions, incomplete combustion of carbon in its numerous forms, and where there is poor ventilation a toxic or lethal concentration may develop. It is present in acetylene, illuminating (coal) gas, furnace and marsh gas, and it is easy to see how a gas which is so prevalent and so readily accessible has played such an important part in the cause of death from poisoning in Great Britain and North America.

Neurological features are common and include abnormal reflexes, increased or diminished, involuntary movements, spasticity and incontinence. If the neurological signs are gross and persist for several days, there is likely to be severe mental impairment when the patient regains consciousness.

The *cerebral pathology* consists of ischaemic changes in the nerve cells with areas of softening in the globus pallidus and cortex. Patients who have residual mental deterioration following the stage of recovery are relatively few in number and are invariably associated with severe intoxication with several days of loss of consciousness.

Mental changes may not follow immediately on exposure and behaviour disturbances may present as long as 21 days afterwards.

Carbon disulphide

This is used extensively in the rubber and rayon industries and prolonged exposure to the chemical can result in mental changes. In the early stages the patient complains of headache, insomnia and bad dreams, and later there is memory loss with intellectual deterioration and occasionally delirium. The neurological symptoms are varied and include tenderness of the nerve trunks, hyperaesthesia and later anaesthesia. Paralysis may ensue and striatal signs with Parkinsonism and choreoathetosis may also occur. There is no effective treatment of the chronic state, though removing the patient from the contaminated area may result in some improvement.

Describe the mental changes due to **internal poisons**

In addition to the failure to eliminate the products of metabolism with consequent toxic effects, disturbance of electrolyte balance may cause mental changes.

Respiratory acidosis

This can be due to a variety of causes, such as depression of the respiratory centre by drugs or disease; weakness or paralysis of the respiratory muscles; reduction of the alveolar area for gaseous exchange, as is seen in pulmonary emphysema, or other pulmonary and cardiac disease; obstruction to the free flow of CO_2 from the lungs, which can be due to either occlusion or severe emphysema;

and breathing an excess of CO_2 as one occasionally finds in closed-circuit anaesthesia where the absorbent is exhausted.

Mental symptoms. These are mainly drowsiness with slow cerebration; the patient may appear demented and occasionally deluded and hallucinated. The condition is liable to exacerbation due to respiratory infection or deterioration in cardiac efficiency and, as cerebral oedema is a complication, the optic discs may suggest increased intracranial pressure. It is not unknown for such patients to be regarded as suffering from brain tumours and to be decompressed. The condition is fairly common in Britain, where chronic bronchitis is prevalent and should be borne in mind, particularly in senile and pre-senile psychotic states.

Treatment. This should be directed to the aetiological factor, though in the severer mental disturbances, phenothiazines may be helpful.

Respiratory alkalosis

This is due to neurotic hyperventilation. The patient may show the signs of tetany with carpal spasm, Chvostek's and Trousseau's signs. There is usually anxiety prior to the attack, but the result of the attack with its threatened loss of consciousness may aggravate the anxiety with resulting panic and occasionally the patient's behaviour can be very disturbing. As many of these patients are in any case very immature, it is difficult to dissociate the behaviour following the hyperventilation from the pre-morbid personality.

Hyponatraemia

This is due to the excessive loss of sodium ion through renal disease, failure of adrenal function, or profuse perspiration. In addition to the fatigue which is common to all causes, in adreno-cortical insufficiency there may be profound depression which can resemble a true psychotic pattern. Occasionally the hypotension and the marked feelings of weakness may earn the patient a diagnosis of neurasthenia. It should therefore be borne in mind in a patient with loss of weight, hypotensive attacks and severe depression, especially as it usually responds to treatment.

Hypokalaemia

Potassium deficit due to either poor intake, as in anorexia nervosa and hyperemesis gravidarum, or excessive loss as in steatorrhoea, can result in mental changes of a delusional or depressive nature. There is also an accompanying confusion, but this may be so slight as to lead the observer to consider the condition to be entirely a functional psychosis. Replacement results in dramatic improvement.

Hypercalcaemia

This may be due to excessive intake of vitamin D, production of some endogenous vitamin D-like substance from sarcoidosis or carcinoma, or increased production of parathyroid hormone from a tumour of the parathyroid glands. Mentally the patient may be apathetic, confused or depressed and present the features of neurasthenia. Surgical removal of the parathyroid tumour usually results in improvement.

Hypocalcaemia

This may follow removal of the parathyroids and the patient will show the clinical features of tetany. His nervous system may be equally irritable, particularly during the attacks of tetany when he may be excitable, restless and confused or present with manic features. Idiopathic hypoparathyroidism could manifest as intellectual deterioration, organic syndrome, functional psychosis or psychoneurosis.

Uraemia

Renal insufficiency results in the retention in the blood of nitrogenous urinary waste products (azotaemia). The causes are many. The main psychiatric interest is in the exclusion of uraemia as a cause of dementia. The patient may be dull, confused and unduly fatigued, and if there is no other obvious cause for the dementia, a blood urea is a useful screening test.

Hepatic coma

This condition is found in liver failure due to disease, drugs, alcohol or following portacaval anastomosis. The patient may present with an encephalopathy with behaviour disturbances, confusion or lethargy. This toxic state is alleged to be caused by an increased concentration of ammonia in the blood due to the inability of the diseased liver to detoxicate it, yet the clinical picture is not highly correlated with the concentration of ammonia in the blood and other metabolites have been considered. The diagnosis is supported by other features of hepatic failure, such as flapping tremor of the hands, spider naevi, and 'liver palms'. EEG changes consisting mainly of generalised slow waves are seen during the attacks.

Mineral metabolism

There is an increasing amount of evidence to show that in people who are apparently physically healthy, psychotic features, particularly mania and melancholia can be associated with fluctuations in sodium when assessed by 'whole-body' techniques. The residual sodium (cell sodium and a small amount of bone sodium) may be increased by 50 per cent in patients with depression and by 200 per cent in patients with mania. Some have attributed the effective use of lithium salts in the treatment of mania as being due to the ability of lithium to substitute for the sodium ion, for when given in therapeutic doses it disturbs sodium transport mechanisms, but the main effect is an exchange of water between the body water compartments.

SECTION 8

PSYCHOSOMATIC MEDICINE

What is a **psychosomatic disorder?**

It is a bodily disorder whose nature can be appreciated only when emotional disturbances (i.e. psychological happenings) are investigated in addition to physical disturbances (i.e. somatic happenings). A 'psychosomatic formula' consists of the following six ingredients:

1. *Emotion as a precipitating factor.* Examination of patients in series shows that in a high proportion of cases, the bodily process emerged or recurred on meeting an emotionally upsetting event.

2. *Personality type.* A particular type of personality appears to be associated with each particular affection.

3. *Sex ratio.* A marked disproportion of sex incidence is a finding in many, perhaps most of these disorders.

4. *Association with other psychosomatic affections.* Different psychosomatic affections may appear in the same individual simultaneously, but the more usual phenomenon as revealed in their natural history is that of the alternation or of the sequence of different affections.

5. *Family history.* A significantly high proportion of cases give a history of the same or an associated disorder in parents, relatives or siblings.

6. *Phasic manifestations.* The course of the illness tends to be phasic with periods of crudescence, intermission and recurrence.

It is not essential for all the ingredients to be present for the condition to merit the label 'psychosomatic'. For example, Nos. 1, 2 or 4 even in isolation would be suggestive and some might include No. 5.

Most languages abound with examples where there is a relationship indicated between emotions and bodily changes, such as 'he gives me a headache', 'the sight of him makes me sick' and 'to die of fright'. A distinction should be drawn between *body*

127

reactions and *body changes* following emotional factors. In the former, the condition is usually regarded as hysterical and denotes a retreat into functional incapacity, such as being struck dumb, blind or paralysed, while in the psychosomatic disorder, overt body changes occur, such as skin rashes, diarrhoea, rectal bleeding and asthmatic attacks.

Cannon's studies on the autonomic system and the bodily changes in pain, hunger and fear provided laboratory confirmation of phenomena which were already well recognised, but more important, they shed some light on how these changes came about. His dictum that sympathetic stimulation prepares the body for fight or flight indicated the importance of the autonomic nervous system and the medulla of the suprarenal glands in these reactions. Experimental evidence of the effect of emotions on the human stomach has been available since Beaumont (1833) studied a patient, Alexis St Martin, who following a gunshot wound of the abdomen had his stomach wall exteriorised. Over 100 years later Wolf and Wolff studied their patient 'Tom', who also had a gastric fistula, and were able to show that gastric secretion, motility and vascularity were reduced when the patient was sad or frightened, but they were increased when he felt angry, resentful or anxious.

Which **theories** *are currently used to describe the physical changes in psychosomatic disorders?*

Selye's theory of the stress-adaptation syndrome

This is based on an adrenocortical response to physical and emotional assaults producing 'stress'. Confirmation of the former is evidenced by the effect of extreme cold, physical trauma, anaesthesia, anoxia, hypoglycaemia and infections, and of the latter by armed combat, boat racing, disturbing interviews, anticipation of surgical operations and final examinations. These are all accompanied by a variable rise in 17-hydroxycorticoid output. The term 'stress' itself has given rise to considerable debate, and in order to understand its place in psychosomatic medicine one should see it under the following four headings:

1. Stress change.
2. Stress situation

3. Stress process.
4. Stress behaviour.

Psychoanalytical theory

The accent of psychoanalysis on oral gratification, habit training, unconscious symbolic use of organs to express conflict and regressive body language or 'organ jargon' has been exploited in the explanation of psychosomatic disorders. These have been listed under the following headings:

1. *Affect equivalents*, where specific physical expressions of any given affect may occur without the corresponding specific mental experiences.
2. *The disturbed chemistry of the unsatisfied person.*
3. *Physical results of unconscious attitudes.* This is elaborated thus: an unusual attitude, which is rooted in unconscious, instinctual conflicts, causes a certain behaviour. This behaviour in turn causes somatic changes in the tissues. The changes are not directly psychogenic; but the person's behaviour, which initiated the changes, was psychogenic.
4. *Hormonal and vegetative dysfunction.* The dictum governing this type of change is, 'every pregenital fixation necessarily changes the hormonal status'.

Psychoanalytic views on psychosexual development have been used to explain some psychosomatic disorders. Oral cravings could colour the personality of the individual who, if approval hungry, would over-react to withdrawal of affection and what has been labelled the 'vital supplies'. The wish to be loved became the wish to be fed, but the wish was not a physiological need, but the result of emotional needs. The stomach could, however, respond as if food were about to be ingested with resulting persistent gastric dysfunction such as chronic hypermotility and hypersecretion with eventual ulcer formation.

Physiological considerations

Experimental work on hypothalamic stimulation with implanted electrodes has been able to produce peptic ulcer in monkeys. Interrelation of the anterior pituitary, adrenal cortex and the vagus as well as the influence of the reticulo-spinal pathways on gastric motility and secretion have been used to explain the genesis of ulcer in physiological terms. (For fuller details see Section 3.)

Discuss the psychiatric aspects of **pain**

Definition. Pain is an unpleasant experience which we primarily associate with tissue damage or describe in terms of tissue damage, or both.

An understanding of the psychological factors which can initiate and exploit pain is dependent on a knowledge of psychological development. This can be summarised thus:

1. *Body image.* It is part of the system which protects the body from injury, in that it warns of damage to or loss of parts of the body. It thus contributes to development of body image and plays a part in the dedifferentiation of the ego.

2. *Object relationships.* Pain in the child provokes crying which elicits comfort from mother and the response is pleasurable. Relief of pain may be equated with reunion with a love object.

3. *Pain and punishment.* These are linked in childhood (as well as semantically). Pain is suffered when child is 'bad' and is therefore deserved and associated with feelings of guilt. It may be cheerfully endured in order to enjoy the forgiveness and reconciliation which follows.

4. *Aggression and power.* The child soon realises he can impose his will by inflicting or threatening pain. He can also control his own aggression by the threat of pain to himself.

5. *Sexual development.* At the height of sexual excitement pain may be mutually inflicted and even enjoyed. Some may prefer the pain to the sexual experience, the latter existing only in phantasy.

What is meant by the **pain-prone?**

In view of the above psychoanalytic interpretation, pain can be used as a psychological means of adjustment, and certain individuals who exploit this mechanism with compulsive repetition are regarded as pain prone. They are generally chronically depressed, pessimistic and gloomy with guilty, self-depreciatory attitudes. They drift into situations or submit to relationships in which they are hurt, beaten, defeated or humiliated, and do not seem to learn from their experience. They often shun success. They seek pain either from their own efforts or at the hands of the physician or surgeon.

Precipitating factors are frequently:

1. Failure of external circumstances to satisfy the unconscious need to suffer.

2. Real, threatened or phantasied loss which may be associated with bereavement.

3. Evocation of guilt by intense aggression or forbidden sexual feelings.

A common precipitating factor in an industrial society is injury. The pain may persist long after the physical effects of the trauma have passed and there are cultural as well as personal factors which mobilise the patient's aggression against the responsible party. It is of interest that if there is no responsible and insured party, persistent pain in industrial injury is rarely seen.

Discuss the psychosomatic disorders associated with the **gastrointestinal** *tract*

Peptic ulcer

The following three conditions are considered to be necessary for the onset of peptic ulcer:

1. A sustained rate of gastric secretion as measured by serum pepsinogen concentration.

2. The presence of a conflict related to the persistence of strong infantile wishes to be loved and cared for, and the repudiation of these wishes by the adult ego or the external world, as inferred from projective and psychological techniques.

3. Exposure to an environmental situation which mobilises conflict and induces psychic tension.

Sex ratio is a contributory factor, and this would fit in with the psychosomatic formula described previously. Stress in the Selye sense has been invoked and it has been demonstrated that peptic ulceration could result from prolonged emotional stress, and this was confirmed during the air-raids in London and Glasgow during the Second World War.

Occupation. There have been differences in incidence amongst various occupations, such as bus drivers as opposed to bus conductors, and this has been attributed to the stressful occupation of driving in a busy city.

Further confirmation of the psychosomatic aspects of peptic ulcer has been shown following gastrectomy where a number of patients break down with either psychiatric illness or alcoholism.

Colitis

'Mucous colitis', 'irritable colon', 'colon neurosis' are terms used to describe a syndrome which in Victorian times was prevalent among parent-dominated, cloistered young women. Psychological factors play a part in either onset or exacerbation. All physical investigations, including biopsy, reveal no abnormality in those patients with the irritable colon. The patient frequently invokes surgery and this insistence used to be gratified, although surgeons are now much more circumspect. Psychiatric treatment in terms of psychotherapy or relaxation can produce useful results, but the personality of the patient may make the condition an intractable one, in that they are often poorly motivated towards recovery.

Discuss the psychiatric aspects of **ulcerative colitis**

A wealth of theorising has been published in relationship to ulcerative colitis, but to date no fully satisfactory hypothesis has been established. Many stress the obsessional and rather rigid and conformist personality of patients with ulcerative colitis and the difficulty they have in overtly expressing their emotions, particularly when in conflict situations which involve loss of a love-object or loss of esteem. It is claimed that when separation cannot be dealt with by the normal psychological mechanisms, such as grief, or by other neurotic or psychotic processes, physiological changes are initiated in the body which interfere with or disrupt other adaptive or integrative processes, thus permitting various types of tissue breakdown, or rendering the tissues susceptible to invasion by viruses or bacteria. Earlier theorists stressed the ejection-riddance pattern involving the large bowel, but this depended on a natural history of ulcerative colitis in which diarrhoea invariably preceded the bleeding. This has however not been substantiated with further studies, and it is clear that when the questions are properly put bleeding is more commonly an early sign than diarrhoea, and therefore any theory will have to take this factor into account. Precipitating factors are extremely common and usually follow stress and school work, marriage and honeymoon, bereavement or leaving home.

A factor which is usually overlooked is that the stress need not necessarily be an unpleasant one and many patients have experienced precipitation or aggravation of their illness following pleasant experiences such as passing examinations, promotion at work or moving into a new house. A high degree of anticipatory excitement such as expecting desirable visitors may also produce a relapse.

Treatment

Engel, who has contributed much to the study of this condition, lays down four basic psychological processes which the doctor must understand before undertaking treatment. These are:

1. The colitic process begins or relapses in a setting in which the patient feels, consciously or unconsciously, that he has suffered or will suffer the loss of an important object relationship.
2. He responds to this with a feeling of helplessness, hopelessness and despair; a feeling that this is 'too much' that he cannot go on.
3. By virtue of a lifelong mutually dependent relationship on certain key figures, especially the mother, he has not achieved the capacity for independent function that characterises the more mature person.
4. He looks to the physician to take over in the areas in which he feels incompetent and not to let him down.

A fifth and obvious rule which tends to be forgotten is that the patient has a very vulnerable colon. Because of the real risk of acute and serious deterioration, the physician who undertakes his treatment should have ready access to a hospital bed, for not only will this add to his confidence in the handling of the patient, but it will also ensure the continuity of treatment and obviate the need to establish too many close personal relationships. Formal analysis is not ruled out as long as the delicacy of the problem is appreciated and there is the closest liaison with the physician, but should there be phases of acute relapse, it would be wise not to subject the patient to further psychotherapy but to retreat to a more supportive role.

Discuss the psychosomatic aspects of the **cardiovascular system**

As with the stomach, the heart has established itself in language as an organ which reflects the emotions and terms like 'heavy heart' and 'light-hearted' are used so freely that their implications may go unrecognised. The heart may be 'sad' or 'merry', 'fickle' or 'sincere', and what is probably a more profound psychological truth, 'in affairs of the heart there is no such thing as reason'. Similarly, the arteries have been implicated, but it is a far cry from metaphor to medicine.

Hypertension

Repressed rage or anger is regarded by some as the principal factor, and if it is not discharged through verbal or motor activity it may take an autonomic and endocrine path which leads to arteriolar constriction and increased peripheral resistance. The precise mechanism has not been satisfactorily demonstrated and the factor of 'the susceptible individual' is an essential constant, but why some should be susceptible in this way is still unknown.

Hypotension

There is stronger evidence of emotional disturbances in hypotension than there is in hypertension. The condition is common and is particularly related to situations involving fear or nausea. In a study of patients in the dental chair, fear was the main cause of hypotension and syncopal attacks, and it has been postulated that emotional stimulation of the heart beat and a fall in cardiac filling pressure may cause virtual emptying of a ventricular chamber during systole which fires the afferent mechanism of the faint reflex.

Coronary artery disease

Studies of pre-morbid personalities have shown that these patients have an intense desire for recognition and are compulsive about time, over-scrupulous and blind to their own limits. They overwork themselves, are unable to relax and feel guilty when trying to do so. Serum cholesterol levels have been studied under situations of stress, such as in students during examinations, or accountants dealing in tax returns, and it is alleged to rise under these circumstances, while the whole blood-clotting time was also accelerated, and these changes were independent of variations in weight, diet and physical activity. When the pressure was lessened, serum cholesterol fell and clotting time returned to normal. Strenuous and unaccustomed exercise is also alleged to be a precipitating factor, and there is a crop of fatalities following a heavy fall of snow with the resultant violent efforts to get the car mobilised. Another factor exists which does not get the same publicity. A common example is when a coronary attack follows the mowing of the lawn. It is frequently associated with remonstrations from the housewife that they are expected elsewhere for tea and he has to wash and change and they will be late. He hurries on and the coronary follows. Another situation is the man with his family on holiday. He is laden with heavy suitcases and there is a train to catch. It would appear that heavy unaccustomed exercise with associated anxiety may be instrumental.

Congestive heart failure

Emotional stress has been blamed for its aggravation or precipitation. Rage, frustration, anxiety, depression or feelings of insecurity have all been regarded as precipitating factors. During such periods of emotional tension or depression, retention of sodium and water has been demonstrated and diuresis follows relaxation of the emotions. Emotions could prove more important than physical activity in determining sodium output, and could be as much as 32 times greater during strenuous activity than during a period of sitting when the patient was tense and anxious. The mechanism is still a matter for speculation, though increased secretion of aldosterone as a result of emotional stress has been postulated to account for the reduced urinary volume and sodium excretion.

Discuss the psychological stresses of **nursing in an intensive care unit**

These are formidable because of the repetitive exposure to death and dying, to the frightening, repulsive and forbidden.

The nurse's psychological experience is one of chronic latent anxiety and tension for though she occupies a place among the hospital's elite, her self-esteem is often threatened, for frequently her patients die, while even her major successes are still usually seriously ill. Attachments are formed to patients and frequent deaths provide a situation of repetitive object-loss.

The intense group loyalty of the unit reinforces work pressure by stimulating guilt about absence from work. The group is self-destructive for it cannot refuse additional work even when the total load is unrealistic, for this would violate group norms and threaten the shared fantasy of omnipotence. The only escape is resignation or flight.

Write a short note on **operant conditioning in heart disease**

Patients with premature ventricular contractions (PVC) have been subjected to operant conditioning which by coloured lights indicated high, low and correct heart rates. After about 10 sessions they were able to increase or decrease the heart rate and maintain it between preset upper and lower limits. They were then able to dispense with the coloured lights and become aware of the PVC through their own sensations. Six elements for successful learning of PVC control are laid down:

1. Peripheral receptors which are stimulated by the PVC.
2. Efferents which carry the information to the CNS.
3. CNS processing to enable the patient to recognize the PVC and to provide the motivation and flexibility necessary for learning to occur.
4. Efferents to an effector organ which can bring about the desired change in the pathologically functioning heart.
5. A heart which is not too diseased to beat more regularly.
6. A homeostatic system in the patient which will tolerate the more normal functioning of the heart.

What psychological factors are associated with **rheumatoid arthritis?**

1. In studies of such patients they usually all present with a diagnosable psychiatric disorder, depression being the commonest.
2. More than half would present or have a history of some other

chronic physical disorder, the commonest being duodenal ulcer, and this was evident prior to treatment with corticoids.

3. These patients do not readily express anger and are over-sensitive.

4. Frequent contacts with the doctor together with drug therapy were more helpful than if the same drug therapy were used, but when consultations were less frequent. Supportive psychotherapy would also enable some patients to progress to the stage where they could overcome repetitive life patterns which would lead them into difficulties.

The presence of an abnormal gamma globulin (rheumatoid factor) in 60-70 per cent of patients has convinced many that the condition is entirely organic. This is not necessarily so, for immune body reactions based on the presence of abnormal gamma globulins could themselves in part be caused by psychological stresses and there is increasing evidence to support this.

Discuss the **psychological aspects of skin disorders**

Statements such as 'the skin is the mirror of the mind' indicate psychological influences on skin conditions. An obvious example is the blush of emotion which may be very difficult to distinguish from the blush of transient erythema or urticaria. In addition there are other aspects of skin diseases which would appear to be associated with psychological factors. For example, the course of a skin disorder, whether it will be acute, sub-acute, chronic, recurrent or intermittent, may well be connected with emotional events in the patient's life. Similarly, skin sensitivity either hyperaesthesia or hyperalgesia which may be demonstrated by a physiologist is frequently closely related to increased skin libidinisation which is described by the psychoanalyst. Also the phenomenon of itching with its attendant rubbing and scratching is frequently associated with neurotic and masochistic overtones.

Describe the **specific skin disorders** which have psychological significance

Itching

It has been shown that tense, anxious or agitated skin patients complain of itching or burning sensations more frequently than the placid, non-anxious and emotionally well integrated.   Further-more, in the same person an unchanged skin lesion would itch more intensely during periods of frustration, boredom or increased tension.   Under psychic stress the wheal and flare produced by an intradermal injection of histamine becomes larger and the ensuing itching more severe and prolonged.

The pleasure derived from scratching can be so intense that it may acquire an auto-erotic quality and be used as a masturbatory substitute.   It can also represent a self-destructive, masochistic action which, besides the dermal pleasure, inflicts punishment and lightens guilt.

These factors are also found in *ano-genital pruritis*, where the psychopathology is similar to that of itching, the patients being usually obsessive-compulsive in nature.

Excessive sweating

Emotional sweating is usually found on palms, soles and axillae, whereas thermal sweating is mostly on the forehead, neck, front and back of the trunk, dorsum of the hand and forearm.   Emotional sweating frequently leads to secondary skin lesions such as vesicula-tion, infections (bacterial and fungal) and rashes.

Alopecia areata

A history of mental shock or acute anxiety frequently precedes the appearance of the bald patches whereas a number exhibit a variety of mental disturbances.

Chronic urticaria

Emotional precipitation is frequently found in such patients and they also show a statistically higher incidence of neurotic symptoms than controls.   Stressful situations are not specific and neither is there a specific personality type.

Atopic dermatitis

The majority of these patients are extremely tense, anxious individuals who are very sensitive to interpersonal contacts.   They are emotionally labile, dependent and hostile, withdrawing easily from unsatisfactory relationships.   Three factors have been associated with this condition:

1. Marked difficulty in expressing aggression and self-assertion.
2. Maternal rejection in childhood, though in some instances there is maternal over-protection.
3. The symptoms frequently have symbolic expressive value as in the case of the man in whom the rash was localised around his wedding ring at a time of marital infidelity.

Urticaria

A relationship between stressful life situations and relapses and exacerbations of the condition have been demonstrated and a regressed aggressiveness and regressed revival of infantile skin eroticism are said to be encountered. Some patients in experimental stress situations may show extreme dilatation of both arterioles and minute vessels, or the cutaneous changes associated with urticaria.

Psoriasis

This disorder affects 1·4 per cent of the population and a recessive gene has been implicated. Non-specific stressful situations may precipitate or aggravate the condition. Pruritis associated with psoriasis is invariably psychogenic and in any patient with this condition investigation of psychiatric factors is essential, especially if showing pronounced fluctuations of symptoms with acute relapses and persistent itching.

Rosacea

This condition and common blushing are said to differ only in degree in that both are emotionally determined. It is occasionally associated with patients with severe depression, and both conditions may clear completely following a course of ECT.

Acne vulgaris and seborrhoeic dermatitis

Although the sebum secretion is not under autonomic control, it may be under humoral control rather than neuronal and stress may well influence the condition. Affective disturbances have been implicated as precipitating factors, and antidepressant agents like imipramine have been reported to effect a remission.

Warts (Verrucae)

These are generally regarded as due to a virus infection but psychological methods are frequently successful in treatment. Suggestion either with or without hypnosis is the commonest method but in patients with depression and tension, the treatment of these conditions can also be helpful.

What is the relationship between **breathing and the emotions?**

Breathing and the emotions are closely related and many novelists have described changes in breathing in order to reinforce the picture of emotional disturbances, particularly in anxiety, passion and rage. The mode of expression is usually pulmonary but on occasions it may be manifest as snorting or sniffing and assume the form of a compulsive act which causes as much if not more distress to the family than to the patient. As respiration has both voluntary and involuntary control, some of its functional disturbances, unlike the stomach and the colon, may be of a voluntary nature, though it should be recognised that this may shade into an involuntary extension.

Describe the **hyperventilation syndrome**

This is found both in children and adults and may be initiated as a voluntary act, though in many instances it is a result of anxiety. It may not be recognised as such, for most do not present with respiratory distress, but with the physical sequelae of the hyperventilation. Some present with cardiovascular symptoms, others, with fainting attacks which may be mistaken for epilepsy, and others with tetany and carpo-pedal spasms. The patient may be in a state of collapse, complaining of precordial pain with pallor, tachycardia, sweating and cold extremities which suggest a recent coronary thrombosis, but the age-group is different, for hyperventilation tends to occur in young people. The washing out of the carbon dioxide leads to vasoconstriction with what has been estimated as a 30 per cent reduction in cerebral blood flow, which may account for the cerebral symptoms. Frequently a complement of phobic anxiety, it is the physical concomitants of the hyperventilation which prevent the patient from overcoming her fears.

Discuss the psychological aspects of **bronchial asthma**

The psychological factors are still debated, and their specificity is still questioned. Comparisons between asthmatic and cardiac children do not show any significant personality differences on psychological tests. Others have claimed that the asthmatic attack is a reaction to the danger of separation from the mother and is the equivalent of an inhibited and repressed cry of anxiety or rage. Psychoanalysts have interpreted the asthmatic attacks as an unconscious attempt by the patient to protect himself from loss of maternal love by respiratory introjection of the ambivalently regarded mother. Unfortunately this does not accord with the clinical features of an asthmatic attack which is not an attempt at respiratory introjection, but difficulty in expiration.

What is the **treatment of bronchial asthma** *with a defined psychosomatic component?*

Psychotherapy has a legitimate place, though as with ulcerative colitis it should be realised that the greatest delicacy in the handling of the patient may be needed, for the condition is likely to, literally, explode in the therapist's face and status asthmaticus is a frightening prospect on the analytical couch. When the mechanism has really got under way, it is virtually impossible to proceed with psychotherapy and too much emphasis on the dynamics of the situation should not blind the therapist to the fact that the patient is exploiting, or is in the grip of, a mechanism which can prove fatal. It is in a spirit of compromise that all therapy must be conducted with the concessions coming mainly from the therapist in the hope that the patient will yield his symptoms.

Hypnosis. Many are convinced of its efficacy while others decry it; some claim it cures, others that it merely relieves the anxiety and permits the condition to subside. It is not essential to prove that hypnosis has a beneficial effect on lung changes to show that it is of value and there is no cause to sneer at a treatment which produces subjective improvement without any physical change. An asthmatic attack is a crippling state and may even prove fatal, so any form of treatment which can either relieve the acute attack or reduce its incidence is of value.

What has been established is that by measuring lung compliance, hypnotic relief of symptoms does not produce any change in lung function so presumably improvement is subjective. Furthermore it is not necessary to induce trance, for many patients would improve in a state which can only be regarded as suggestion under relaxation, and it may be that the relief of anxiety in those patients who already have organic changes in their lungs lowers the demands on a failing respiratory system by lowering the basal metabolic rate. Hypnosis can also be effective in some cases of status asthmaticus.

What is **psychogenic dyspnoea?**

This is a condition where the respiratory distress is disproportionate to the patient's airways obstruction. When such patients are compared with a control group the following factors have been defined: (1) poor relationship of breathlessness to exertion; (2) acute hyperventilation attacks present; (3) breathlessness experienced at rest; (4) main difficulty was getting air in; (5) breathlessness fluctuated even in minutes; (6) fear sudden death in attack of hyperventilation; (7) breathlessness varied with social situation; (8) patient had stopped working; (9) not improved by stopping smoking; (10) breathless during conversation; (11) relieved by sedatives and alcohol; (12) woken at night by breathlessness; (13) worse in the morning and evening and not relieved by expectoration.

Successful treatment of the accompanying psychiatric disorder, usually depression or an anxiety state, can result in a total or partial resolution of breathlessness.

Write short notes on the psychosomatic aspects of:

1. **Bronchial carcinoma**

As with many patients with psychosomatic disorders, these patients have been described as having a poor outlet for emotional discharge. More evidence is accumulating to indicate that cancer of the lung does occur in people with certain backgrounds and personalities, and this is in accord with other studies of certain forms of cancer. More information is however awaited before any firm conclusions can be drawn.

2. Allergic rhinitis

This frequently has a psychological component. The nose has been regarded as symbolic of the sexual organ and it is considered that repressed olfactory sexual curiosity may play a part, the patient having substituted the olfactory organ for the visual one. At a more superficial level, the condition is in some people a distress signal and may appear on specific occasions, such as when making an after-dinner speech or presenting a paper to a learned society.

3. The common cold

Some people are much more prone than others to this condition and the possibility of psychological factors has been raised. Children who are prone to these colds frequently fit into the category of the nervous child and are prone not only to the common cold but other respiratory tract infections. They frequently come from broken homes and those who were attending nursery schools had a significantly higher number of absences which were alleged to be due to colds than those from better homes.

4. Pulmonary tuberculosis

The psychological aspects of this condition have long interested the physician and the phenomenon of *spes phthisica* where the patient is unduly euphoric has been associated with underlying instability. Those who deal with these patients have frequently remarked on the difficulties some have in responding to effective treatment and put this down to lowered resistance which could have psychological causes. Such patients are healthy bodied, live in comfortable material circumstances and the only factors which can be determined are psychological ones. Some have found that the disease is commonest in patients with an inordinate need for affection and the commonest emotional factor preceding the onset in these patients was a break in a love link, such as romance, engagement or marriage.

What are the psychological factors associated with obesity?

It has been regarded as an organ neurosis exhibiting oral gratification with emotional immaturity and undue dependence on the 'vital supplies'. It has been pointed out that the child may go in for the pleasures of food if he does not get the pleasure of love from his parents. The usual traumatic experiences are withdrawal or threatened withdrawal of affection and the patient then regresses to an earlier oral erotic level where oral gratification is used to create a feeling of security. The rapid increase in weight in those who give up smoking has also been explained on this basis.

Sudden obesity may follow psychological trauma and precipitating factors may be the death of a mother, an unwanted pregnancy or the hazard of an air-raid. Obesity is therefore evidence of underlying instability which can manifest in other ways, such as drug addiction, alcoholism, depression and phobic anxiety.

What is meant by the **night-eating syndrome?**

This is manifested usually with noctural hyperphagia, insomnia and morning anorexia. It is usually evidenced during periods of weight gain and increased stress. A reducing regime with weight loss may result in depression and anxiety.

Discuss psychogenic **polydipsia and polyuria**

These used to be confused with diabetes insipidus and some of the tests such as the administration of nicotine or hypertonic saline and dehydration may be unreliable and even dangerous. A test which is alleged to be more reliable and safer is that of withholding water for six and a half hours and taking samples of serum and urine at the beginning, middle and end of the period. The psychogenic group show a greater ratio of urine to serum osmolarity than any of the patients with known diabetes insipidus, particularly in the last hour of the test. Psychogenic polydipsia is usually associated with obesity for the preferred drinks are frequently sweetened fruit-juices. This obesity itself may suggest an organic diagnosis as it is often regarded as convincing evidence of hypothalamic involvement.

What is meant by **psychogenic fever?**

Habitual hyperthermia in young women has been demonstrated, particularly in those who are neurotic with no evidence of organic disease. It has frequently been attributed to anxiety or tension and discussion of the patient's problem with a solution of the difficulties may result in a defervescence. Many patients with psychogenic fever suffer from other psychosomatic disorders.

Discuss the psychosomatic aspects of **pregnancy**

During pregnancy old unconscious phantasies are mobilised. These are associated with introjection and women with oral fixations and ambivalent attitudes to their pregnancy will revive old conflicts associated with oral strivings. The food cravings of pregnant women have been studied but physiological interpretations have not been substantiated, and it is now generally agreed that they are primarily psychological. Sometimes the craving is for fruit, vegetables and non-food substances, such as coal, soap, disinfectant, and there are also aversions such as to tea, tobacco and coffee. These cravings are commoner in the first four months of pregnancy and rarely persist the full term. Sometimes it is the texture of the material rather than the flavour which is desired, and among food cravings are pickled foods, nuts, dry, raw cereal and uncooked vegetables. A number admit to pica.

Discuss the psychological aspects of **dyspareunia**

It has been explained as a defence against sexual intercourse, which in turn may be based on phantasies of injury. Although analytical treatment has been favoured, simpler methods such as reassurance can be just as effective and much speedier. Explanatory talks with the emphasis on the importance of relaxation are usually successful, and occasionally dilatation either with finger or with a glass dilator is necessary.

Is **hyperemesis gravidarum** a psychosomatic disorder?

Many of the studies of this problem are based either on the personality of the patient or on psychological factors which may have affected the patient's attitude to the pregnancy. Conflicting reports have resulted in that some regard it as not having any psychological overtones while others are quite satisfied that it is definitely a psychosomatic disorder.

It can be a very serious disability and patients have been at the point of death with marked ketosis and termination of pregnancy used to be not infrequent. Now the situation is much more hopeful in that the electrolyte depletion can be replaced and incidentally the mental state of the patient which may have resulted from this is speedily corrected and the patient's co-operation can be insured. The problem frequently becomes an issue between the patient and the nursing staff, and the doctor's role may be that of explaining the problem to the nursing staff in order to create a more favourable climate for the patient. The problem is now not nearly as grave as it used to be and extreme cases rarely present although the milder cases must still be very common.

Discuss the psychiatric disorders of pregnancy

These are mainly post-partum though in a few instances they may appear during pregnancy. The incidence of the severer forms is not more than 1 per 800-1000 live births though milder forms are commoner. Although they are frequently referred to as *puerperal psychoses*, most occur between the 6th and 12th weeks after delivery. They are generally unpredictable though patients with a previous history of puerperal psychosis or other mental illness or with a family history of mental illness are more vulnerable but not sufficiently so to predict the occurrence with any accuracy. All attempts to define an endocrinological cause for the condition have, to date, been unsuccessful.

Clinical features

These are mainly manic, depressive, schizo-affective or frankly schizophrenic. While it is possible for a woman suffering from a psychosis to become pregnant, the illness is not usually aggravated by pregnancy, rather the reverse. The vast majority of puerperal psychoses come 'out of the blue' and frequently develop rapidly. This is seen particularly in mania which is the one variety which usually occurs in the strict puerperium. In a matter of hours a quiet patient can be literally 'crawling up the wall'. The other reactions can also be very marked with florid delusional features and suicide is a major hazard.

Treatment. The manic states can generally be brought rapidly under control with haloperidol 5 mg. t.d.s. coupled with Benzhexol 2 mg. t.d.s. to counter striatal side-effects. It is important to maintain the control for several weeks, at least, for the condition may still be active and relapse is likely.

The depressive, schizo-affective and schizophrenic varieties, if severe, should be treated with ECT for they generally respond quickly. Conservative treatment will suffice in the less severe and will consist of effective tricyclics and if necessary major tranquillizers. Much has been made of admitting the baby to hospital with the mother but many years of ,observation of this method and of treating the mother apart has not proved that one method is superior to the other. Much will depend on the individual circumstances and there will be instances where it is necessary to separate mother from child.

What psychological aspects are associated with **urinary retention?**

This is a common condition post-operatively and functional factors predominate. It is seen most commonly, as one would expect, after gynaecological surgery or operations on the urinary tract. It may also follow childbirth, marital discord and broken love-affairs. Successful treatment by psychotherapy has been reported, and in the exploration of these patients there have been histories of sexual traumas, seduction and rape. In some instances it may be used as a means of reinforcing a frigidity and fear of sexual intercourse.

Discuss **pre-menstrual tension and dysmenorrhoea**

In addition to the tension there is irritability and depression in the pre-menstrual phase and there may be evidence of water retention such as swelling of the breasts and abdomen and even frank oedema. Other psychosomatic components associated with the condition are higher accident rate, increased incidence of suicide, increase in misbehaviour and crime, and acute psychiatric illness. The evidence of fluid retention as a factor has not been universally agreed and some investigators have been unable to find any response to chlorothiazide, while others regard the functional element as a dominant one. This was reinforced by a clinical trial comparing meprobamate and chlorothiazide in the treatment of the condition, in which the former achieved a much higher rate of success.

Other benzodiazepines such as diazepam, lorazepam and medazepam have been found helpful, though there is always a slight risk of addiction.

Dysmenorrhoea is said to occur in anxious or hostile women who reject their feminine role but the evidence is mainly derived from individual patients undergoing psycho-analysis. It would be too big a step to explain the vast numbers who suffer from dysmenorrhoea on this basis. Much of the symptomatology is tied up with the experience of pain and pain thresholds.

What are the psychiatric sequelae of abortion and sterilisation?

Abortion which is frequently advised on psychiatric grounds has its own psychiatric hazards. In Ekblad's series of 479 patients, 11 per cent had material psychiatric disturbance and 25 per cent regretted the operation. Generally, the more unstable the patient, the greater the psychiatric hazards of abortion. The clinical condition is usually depression though schizophrenic reactions may also occur. Prognosis is not as good as with post-puerperal psychoses.

Ekblad described similar psychiatric sequelae following sterilisation and came to the same conclusion, viz. that the more unstable the patient, the more adverse would be her response to the operation. These findings are not universal and it may be because 98 per cent of Ekblad's sterilisations had an abortion as part of a 'package deal'. In clinics where abortion was not advised and the sterilisation either followed delivery or was undertaken independently of pregnancy, there has been very little in the way of psychiatric sequelae.

Discuss the psychosomatic aspects of vasectomy *and* sterilisation

In the former, most subjects and their wives react as if the operation had demasculating potential with resulting psychological upset. Such reactions may be reduced by full discussion prior to the operation. It is recommended that applicants be screened for pre-existing instability.

In the latter, adverse effects may also ensue and the following criteria have been suggested:

1. The patient should be over the age of 30, and if younger should have had two or more children.

2. The operation should not be performed at childbirth or in the neonatal period, when the risk to the newborn child is greatest. Sterilisation could, with the death of the child, compound the loss and precipitate a severe grief reaction. Furthermore, the mother's decision at that time may not be as valid a one as she may make three to six months later.

3. The patient should not be suffering from a postabortive depression, for a sterilisation may reinforce this reaction.

4. The patient should be culturally adjusted to the operation.

5. The operation should not be undertaken for frigidity.

6. Apart from conclusion 3, psychiatric considerations need not be entertained.

7. It should not be part of a 'package deal' as a condition for an abortion.

What evidence is there of **psychological factors in infertility?**

Infertility is frequently associated with stress and particularly a disturbance in the marital relations. Of the mechanisms involved, it has been shown that emotional shock can produce an immediate effect on the endometrium, while emotional immaturity may be associated with tubal spasm and the presence of hypogonadal genitalia. Some immature, infertile women have bacterial infection of the cervical mucus which clears up with their emotional problems. Many have a dry cervix with scanty, sticky mucus associated with hypogonadism and the mucus may be related to chronic pelvic congestion due to regular sexual stimulation without satisfaction.

Tubal spasms may be associated with tension as well as general immaturity and when testing for tubal patency the patient should be conscious for the spasm may disappear under the anaesthetic. Adoption may also facilitate conception by relieving emotional stress.

What psychosomatic factors can be identified with **migraine?**

Migraine is frequently held to represent an inborn type of

reaction to a number of stresses, both psychological and physical, and although psychological factors may precipitate an attack, many neurologists are reluctant to accept the fact that migraine is a psychogenic affection curable by psychotherapy. The explanation for the discrepancy between the psychiatrist's attitude and the neurologist's attitude is that they may well be seeing different aspects of the problem. The neurologist frequently sees a patient with migraine with a neurological lesion, while the psychiatrist has the patient 'filtered' for him and is sent migrainous conditions which have no neurological basis. Another adulterating factor is that ordinary headaches are frequently equated with migraine, particularly in certain cultures, and headaches are notoriously associated with abnormal personality responses, such as conversion hysteria and hypochondriasis.

Discuss the psychosomatic aspects of **anorexia nervosa**

The name was originally coined by Gull (1874). It is traditionally seen in young adolescent girls, though anorexia may also be a feature of psychiatric disorders such as severe depression and schizophrenia as well as a manifestation of a paranoid state, the patient refusing food because of some delusion, for example, that he is being poisoned. The condition varies in severity and many are seen by family doctors and only a small number have to be admitted to hospital.

Psychopathology. This is mainly concerned with the patient's oral drives. Refusal to eat in children may be used to express negative feelings toward the parents. The offer of food by a parent to a child has a symbolic meaning, for it represents love, and some parents who feel insecure can only appreciate an acceptance and reciprocation of their love in the child's appetite. The condition is usually seen in girls and in a family situation where the child conflicts with the mother or where the father is dominant. The girl will cleave to the father and may try to usurp the mother's place by various devices such as following the father's occupation.

In addition to the anorexia nervosa there is frequently a disturbance in body image, the concept reaching delusional proportions. Psychoanalytic treatment is generally ineffective and management of the case is the most certain way to avert disaster which may result in death.

Endocrine factors. Although a search for these has been persistent, nothing has yet emerged and there is no evidence to suggest that the condition is other than a functional one.

Clinical features. The patient is usually a young unmarried girl of good or average intelligence whose behaviour in other respects has hitherto been impeccable. She is usually conscientious, with a high moral code and a flair for doing good and may be a member of voluntary organisations like the Red Cross or Girl Guides, and may even hold office. There is often a history of fluctuation in weight, the patient putting on and taking off weight with the speed of a prize-fighter and the obesity is no less evidence of the underlying instability than the anorexia.

The home environment is usually very sympathetic but ineffective in dealing with the problem and the mother may very readily be caught up in the patient's ideas on feeding, ministering small sips of a low-calorie meat essence to a girl who is dangerously emaciated, or even reinforce the patient's refusal to come into hospital. All forms of subterfuge may be used to get rid of food and these patients become most expert in disposing of it. The patient may have an air of brightness and sparkle and appear energetic, going to work and showing her usual zest and enthusiasm and compensating for any anaemia with lavish applications of make-up. Some have delusional aspects *re* the body image, insisting that they are overweight, indulge in mirror-gazing and keep displaying their scaphoid abdomens to prove their argument. Others develop food fads, but these exclude the nutritious varieties and may be mainly for watery fruits such as melons. A number are prone to shoplifting, particularly from food stores. It can also occur in males.

Physically the gross emaciation may be camouflaged with clothing. A fine lanugo-like hair covers the body. Amenorrhoea is universal, and the B.M.R. is reduced considerably.

Treatment. In the milder cases this can be psychotherapeutic. Phantasies *re* oral impregnation can be discussed and in certain instances a more analytical approach with efforts to deal with the unresolved oedipal situation may be attempted. In hospital these patients are adept at handling mother substitutes, and the ward sister is particularly vulnerable. The doctor is the father-figure, and the patient is likely to recreate the home situation.

F

Management. Regular weighing at not more than three-day intervals should be carried out, for a week may be too long and provide the shock of a substantial loss of weight. Strict nursing supervision with an attitude of benevolent neutrality is a good policy under which the patient's anxiety gradually settles. Over-optimism is the cardinal error in treatment and the patient should be nursed in bed with cot-sides up, taken to and from the toilet and allowed to sit up only under supervision. Like alcoholism, one lapse is invariably the precursor of rapid deterioration and it should not be ignored. Some favour tube feeding, and this may be necessary in extreme cases. The most useful pharmacological measure is chlorpromazine in large doses, which lowers the patient's active resistance and makes them more amenable to nursing attention. Modified insulin is often used as an adjunct.

Discuss the psychosomatic aspects of **hyperuricaemia**

As many sufferers from gout have been men of distinction and the disease tends to occur in patients from the higher social classes, there is a tendency to equate high serum levels of uric acid with social and economic success. Higher than average levels of uric acid were most closely associated with the personal characteristics of drive, achievement and leadership. Other correlates were obesity, alcohol consumption and a good appetite.

Discuss the **psychogenesis of organic disease**

It is now being advocated that a number of organic diseases, some of which are fatal, may be initiated by psychological factors. Experimental evidence of this has come from animals, such as wild rats, who when their whiskers were cut off and they were deprived of their customary reassuring sensory input would have a cardiac arrest in diastole when exposed to a frightening experience. Engel has put forward the concept of the *withdrawal-conservation* response to certain stresses where the organism prepares not for fight or flight but for depletion and exhaustion, and this has also been called the *giving in* syndrome. This has been alleged to play a part in the development of cancer, and other conditions such as autoimmune diseases.

List other diseases where psychosomatic factors have been shown to operate

Multiple sclerosis has been precipitated by (a) sudden threat to patient's own life or to the life of an important object; (b) recent object loss by death; (c) removal of body parts or iatrogenic changes in body function; (d) significant events in the family; (e) family conflicts; (f) graduation or promotion; (g) planned or actual marriage or parenthood.

Behçet's syndrome. These patients tend to be excessively dependent on spouse or parents, are over-submissive and communicate hostility indirectly. Severe relapses are frequently related to life situations where reality demands cannot be tolerated.

Chronic prostatitis. Patients who do not respond to treatment are generally anxious with feelings of guilt and self-reproach concerning their illness which they view as punishment. They frequently become addicted to prostatic massage.

Haemophilia. Many of these boys who take part in strenuous games and sports such as boxing and football do not bleed profusely when injured, yet a gentle knock in a similar area under different circumstances could produce a severe haemorrhage.

What is the expectation of life among widowers?

In a follow-up of such patients of 55 years of age or older over a 9-year period, there was a mortality rate during the first 6 months of bereavement which was 40 per cent above the expected rate for married men of the same age. Thereafter the rate gradually fell to that of married men. The commonest cause was coronary thrombosis and other arteriosclerotic and degenerative heart disease.

SECTION 9

AFFECTIVE DISORDERS

What is meant by **affect and affective disorders?**

Affect is a term used for the emotional or feeling aspect of mental life, or mood.

Affective disorders refer to mental illnesses where the predominant abnormality is a disturbance of affect; these include various forms of depression, and mania.

Give an outline of the classification and clinical features of **depressive illnesses**

Depressions have often been classified on the basis of aetiology, e.g. reactive if produced by environmental stresses and endogenous if no precipitating factor can be demonstrated and the depression is thought to arise 'from within', perhaps on a genetic basis. However, it is generally accepted that a full delineation of the aetiology is frequently impossible and a description of the clinical syndrome is more meaningful. Further, it has been shown that in the majority of so-called 'endogenous' depressions, a precipitating factor can be elicited.

Depressions are usually divided into:

1. *Neurotic.*
2. *Psychotic.* This group includes depression occurring in manic-depressive states, and 'involutional depression'.

(The entity of *reactive* depression signifies the occurrence of a depressive illness in a stable personality as the result of overwhelming stress; hence it is relatively rare.)

The clinical features of both groups may display depressed mood, tearfulness, inability to concentrate, general lack of interest, insomnia, poor appetite, preoccupation with bodily health (hypochondriasis), irritability, diminished libido and feelings of strangeness or unreality (depersonalisation). Similarly, in depression of some severity, suicidal ideas may emerge.

The following features help to *distinguish psychotic from neurotic depression:*

1. *History*

The patient with psychotic depression might give a history of previous, similar depressions, or an attack of mania, with full recovery between the episodes of illness. The neurotic depressive is likely to give a history of several depressive episodes, always precipitated by stress, although the stress may well have been relatively trivial in nature. There may also be a history of previous overt neurosis, e.g. anxiety state, obsessional neurosis or hysterical behaviour.

2. *Family history*

The family of a psychotic depressive may produce a positive psychiatric history, e.g. of depression, mania or suicide.

3. *Personality*

The patient with a psychotic depression may have a cyclothymic (mood-swinging) premorbid personality, or a hypothymic one (tendency to be somewhat depressed), but will have been fairly effective in the past. The neurotic depressive tends to have a vulnerable or inadequate type of personality, or exhibits features of neuroticism. An anxious, hysterical or obsessional premorbid personality may be found.

4. *Precipitating factors*

It is often said that neurotic depressions are 'understandable' or 'justifiable', whereas psychotic depressions tend to come 'out of the blue'. Most psychotic depressions have precipitating factors too, but relationship is less 'justifiable' for it may follow an illness like 'flu or a trivial incident, particularly involving the loss or threatened loss of a love object. A history is often obtained that the patient has overworked and exhausted himself immediately prior to succumbing to a depressive illness. This can be erroneously attributed to the overwork, but the overwork may be symptomatic of a mild hypomanic episode which has preceded the onset of the depression.

5. *Symptoms*

(*a*) Anxiety symptoms are more common in neurotic depression, as is also the type of insomnia seen in neurotic patients, viz. difficulty in getting off to sleep.

(*b*) Early morning waking is seen especially in psychotic depression.

(*c*) Diurnal variation. In psychotic depression, the patient tends to be at his worst in the morning, improving as the day progresses; in neurotic depression, the reverse trend tends to be the case, with worsening as the day goes on.

(*d*) Although hypochondriasis occurs in both types of depression, it usually has a distinctly neurotic flavour in the patient with neurotic depression, i.e. the somatic complaints are multiple, may vary from day to day, affect different systems of the body, and are paraded in an attention-seeking manner; in addition the degree of hypochondriasis flunctuates considerably. In the psychotic depressive, hypochondriacal ideas usually focus on one organ or system, are tenaciously and consistently held, and may assume delusional intensity, e.g. the patient may actually believe that he has cancer and is going to die.

(*e*) The following features occur only in the psychotic type of depression:

Delusions by definition are psychotic features. Hypochondriacal delusions occur, but also delusions of guilt; the patient may believe himself guilty of some crime; he may have a very low opinion of himself, be self-deprecatory, condemnatory and reproach himself for imaginary misdeeds. The delusions may be nihilistic (there being nothing left in life) or of poverty. The patient may project his feelings on to others and feel persecuted, or be subject to ideas of reference.

Hallucinations, like delusions, when present, are in keeping with the depressive affect. The patient may have auditory hallucinations, e.g. hearing voices mocking him or plotting against him, or olfactory hallucinations, perceiving foul odours emanating from him.

Retardation, a general slowing of mental as well as of motor activity tends to occur only in psychotic depression. and when extreme is called *stupor*. Physiological sluggishness such as bradycardia, low blood pressure, dryness of mucous membranes and constipation is more commonly associated with psychotic depression.

Other forms of depression

1. Mixed type, where both neurotic and psychotic forms occur in the same patient.
2. Secondary ('symptomatic') depression. Here the depression is the expression of an underlying physical illness. Common causes are cerebral tumour, early dementia, myxoedema and malignant disease. In the last, depression may appear before the primary lesion has declared. Other associated conditions are epilepsy, alcoholism and schizophrenia.
3. Schizo-affective illness.

Discuss the aetiology of depression

1. *Heredity*

Manic-depressives (*bipolar*) bear a stronger genetic predisposition than depressives (unipolar). Familial incidence, which is very common, does not necessarily implicate heredity, but often connotes environmental and sub-cultural influences.

2. *Constitution*

A 'pyknic' body habitus is commonly found in manic-depressives, and in cyclothymics.

3. *Personality*

A cyclothymic personality is common in manic-depressives but the premorbid personality of depressives is more varied.

4. *Neurophysiology*

Disturbances in the diencephalic-limbic systems can produce mood changes, especially depression—while temporal lobe epilepsy and prefrontal leucotomy can produce alterations in affect.

5. *Biochemistry*

(*a*) Sodium and water retention have been demonstrated in mania and to a lesser extent in psychotic depression. Hormone secretion from the adrenal cortex is altered in severe depression with a raised plasma cortisol as well as dysfunction of the pituitary-adrenal axis. The latter can be reflected in abnormality in dexamethasone-suppression. A further biochemical upset often demonstrable in severe depression is increased resistance to insulin-induced hypoglycaemia.

(b) Catecholamine hypothesis. This proposes that many depressions are associated with a deficiency of catecholamines, especially noradrenaline, at functionally important adrenergic receptor sites in the brain. Conversely, elation or mania may be associated with an excess of such amines. The hypothesis derives from the chemical action of the antidepressant drugs, which increase brain catecholamines with potentiation of noradrenaline activity in animals. Furthermore, reserpine which produces depression in animals and man, depletes brain stores of serotonin and noradrenaline. These corticoids tend to divert amines along the kynurenine pathway away from the noradrenaline one.

More recently research has paid attention to the varying qualities and properties of brain amines and the ways in which they act at different receptor sites. In this alternative theory, certain brain amines such as serotonin are designated 'Type B amines' and are thought to be biphasic, i.e. able to act both on excitant and depressant receptors.

Serotonin has thus also been implicated in amine theories. Tryptamine excretion has been found to be reduced in severe depression often rising to normal levels as recovery occurs. Also, 5HIAA, a metabolite of serotonin, has been found to be low in the cerebrospinal fluid of depressives.

6. Psychopathology

Psychoanalytic theory maintains that loss of self-esteem or of a love object are often involved in depression. Similarly, hypochondriasis and psychotic depression are explained as a narcissistic regression, consisting of a withdrawal of libido from object relationships. Another hypothesis is that depressives (neurotic and psychotic) are approval hungry, and withdrawal or the threat of it may precipitate a depression.

7. *Physiological changes*

These are seen especially in psychotic forms of depression, and occur most constantly in patients who are retarded (*vide supra*). Salivary rates, blood flow in muscles and sweat gland activity have all been studied in such patients, and have been associated with a general reduction.

Precipitating factors

Most depressions are preceded by physical or psychological stress factors. Also, an attack of hypomania may come before the depression sets in. The common precipitating factors are:

(*a*) *Physical.* Infections, e.g. influenza, infective hepatitis, glandular fever. Operations, accidents, endocrine changes, e.g. pregnancy, childbirth, menopause and endocrine disease, e.g. hypo- and hyperthyroidism. Drugs, e.g. those used in the treatment of hypertension such as reserpine, methyl dopa and clonidine, corticosteroid preparations and contraceptive pills.

Chronic illness of any type may be relevant, especially if acting in combination with social isolation. This is seen especially in elderly patients, where psychological factors such as retirement, loss of spouse or altered circumstances may also be operating.

(*b*) *Psychological.* Some form of loss or disappointment is the most frequent theme. Withdrawal of affection, damage to self-esteem, bereavement and moving house are common factors in this category.

Outline the **treatment of depressive illnesses**

1. *Environmental stresses*

If these are defined in the aetiology an attempt should be made to deal with them. This may involve giving attention to home or work situation. Home visits by social workers may be helpful both in assessing these stresses as well as the relatives' attitudes, and in effecting desirable changes. These factors are mainly operative in the neurotic type of depression.

2. *Psychotherapy*

Supportive psychotherapy may be useful as one of the lines of treatment in any depressive illness. Neurotic depressives often have vulnerable or frankly unstable personalities, if not overt neuroses, and require, in addition to physical methods of treatment, some psychological help in general adaptation. Where the premorbid personality is good, simple supportive psychotherapy plus antidepressant drugs usually produces good results.

The patient with psychotic depression might require reassurance, e.g. with regard to his feelings of guilt, unworthiness and hopelessness, but intensive psychotherapy is contraindicated, since this often leads to intensification of the patient's ideas of guilt, with an attendant risk of suicide.

3. *Antidepressant drugs*

Either the tricyclic or monoamine oxidase inhibitor group of antidepressants may be used in treatment of a depressive illness, although the former have less undesirable side-effects. Some claim that the MAOI are more useful in the treatment of neurotic depression, whereas the tricyclic group are indicated in the psychotic (or endogenous) forms of depression.

4. *Other drugs*

In the restless or agitated patient, tranquillisers, e.g. phenothiazines or benzdiazepines, may be useful.

5. *Electroconvulsive therapy* (ECT)

This very useful treatment is indicated in the more severe forms of psychotic depression, viz, where ideas (or delusions) of guilt, intense feelings of self-reproach or suicidal thoughts are present, or when the patient exhibits retardation or stupor. In the patient who is severely retarded and is not eating, the administration of ECT may be life-saving. The treatment has few contraindications, and these include severe cardio-pulmonary disease, e.g. recent myocardial infarction, and organic brain disease. Unilateral ECT (see Section 18) is sometimes used, since there is some evidence that subsequent memory disturbance is minimised.

6. *Prefrontal leucotomy*

This operation is reserved for the patient who suffers from repeated attacks of psychotic depression, where more conservative methods of treatment are no longer effective. The operation should be restricted to those who fulfil, in addition, the following criteria: good premorbid personality; anxiety or tension. A supportive home environment is essential, since post-leucotomy progress is influenced to a large extent by rehabilitation.

Write notes on **suicide and attempted suicide**

Suicide rate in England and Wales is approximately 11 per 100,000 of the population. The suicide rate is a rather crude statistic, however, being dependent on the verdicts of coroners' inquests. In the average general practice there will be, roughly, one suicide every three years.

The following factors appear to be important:

1. Social isolation. Suicide rates tend to be higher in areas of social disorganisation and in the bedsitter-lodging house areas of large cities. Loneliness and loss of feelings of identity with the social group are probably relevant. There is a higher rate among immigrants.

2. Age and sex. The elderly have the highest suicide rate per unit of population at risk; commoner in males.

3. Social class. Suicide rates are highest among the upper social classes.

4. Season. Suicide in Europe is commoner in the spring.

5. Mental or physical illness frequently antedates the suicide act. Ninety per cent of suicides have been suffering from a mental disorder, psychotic depression and alcoholism being the most relevant here. Up to 25 per cent of suicides have suffered from some form of physical illness and the majority have been in touch with their family doctor or with a hospital out-patient clinic in the preceding month.

6. Method. Coal-gas poisoning was for many years the most frequently employed method of suicide, but with detoxication of domestic gas supplies, drug overdosage has gone from second place to top of the league. Hanging, drowning, shooting are less common.

Theories of suicide include:

1. Durkheim—loss of identity with social group.
2. *Psychoanalytic*

Freud—the death instinct ('thanatos') may express itself in the suicidal act. The central theme of all the psychoanalytic views on suicide is that of aggression, viz. the punitive and self-destructive drives, but are also directed outwards, at a person whom the suicide either hates or to whom he is ambivalent.

Menninger states that in suicide, three elements are usually present in varying degree, viz. the desire to kill, to be killed and to die.

Attempted suicide. This term, although popularly employed, is in fact inaccurate, since the majority of patients who make a suicidal gesture such as taking an overdose of drugs are not really intent on suicide. These acts of 'attempted suicide' or 'self-poisoning' (where drugs are ingested) occur nine times more frequently than actual suicide. In the average general practice roughly three patients per year make some such attempt. Of those who make suicide attempts about 1 per cent will be successful in a subsequent attempt within one year.

'Attempted suicide' is quite different from suicide, and tends to occur in a different type of person in different types of circumstances, although there is a little overlap in those mentally ill. Many so-called 'suicidal attempts' are in the nature of a cry for help, or attempt to deal with a distressing personal situation, such as a troubled relationship with someone else, or difficulties over money, housing, etc. Sometimes this act is impulsive, e.g. after a quarrel. Occasionally, self-poisoning may be accidental, e.g. the taking of too many sleeping tablets because of an intolerance of insomnia.

Self-poisoning is increasing, and it is likely that social and cultural influences and availability of drugs are relevant.

Other factors associated with attempted suicide include:

1. Sex. More frequently in females.
2. Age. Commonly seen in younger age-groups, viz. adolescents and young adults.
3. Marital status. High prevalence of the unmarried, separated and divorced.

4. Social isolation. Not so important a factor as in suicide proper, but sometimes seen because of recent break-up of relationship.

5. Financial problems. Sudden reduction in income more important than poverty.

6. Alcoholism. Commonly observed (up to 20 per cent). Drug abuse is a common feature in younger age groups.

7. Family background. Broken homes or other evidence of deprived childhood frequently observed.

8. Previous history: (a) mental illness or instability in about 50 per cent; (b) previous suicidal attempt in about 20 per cent; (c) a criminal record in males who attempt suicide is more common than in the general population.

Who are the Samaritans?

It is an organisation comprised mainly of voluntary workers whose aim is to answer distress calls from those who feel at risk of committing suicide. Such potentially suicidal people are able to telephone the local Samaritans and obtain immediate help and advice and the organisation has spread to many parts of the country. The majority of the clientele consist of the lonely and the unstable. Attempts are now being made to evaluate the Samaritans in relation to their effect, if any, on the suicide rate. There are comparable groups in the U.S.A., usually called 'Suicide Prevention' Services.

Define mania and hypomania

Mania is an affective disorder characterised by elated mood, rapid speech and general overactivity. The illness is often accompanied by grandiose delusions, and, like psychotic depression, is usually classified under the 'functional psychoses'. Patients who have a constitutional predisposition (probably genetically determined) to develop mania often have a tendency to develop psychotic depression, and are regarded as 'manic-depressives'. It is said to be commoner in females.

Hypomania has the same characteristics as mania, but the illness is less severe.

Mania and hypomania occur mainly in people of cyclothymic

personality, i.e. those subject to extreme swings of mood, and like depression it is often precipitated by physical illness, including brain disease.

Describe the **symptomatology** of mania

1. *Onset.* It may follow a period of extreme well-being, or a depressive illness. It may also occur during the treatment of depression, the patient 'spilling over' from a remission.

2. *Prodromal features.* The patient requires less sleep and becomes more active generally, taking on extra work and responsibilities; he is generally euphoric and very energetic. He becomes excessively optimistic and this may lead a business-man or professional man to undertake heroic schemes which alarm his colleagues. At this stage, he may be very irritable.

3. *Activity.* All behaviour is characterised by overactivity. This may manifest itself as excessive letter writing or the display of an abnormal amount of energy with marked restlessness.

4. *Mood.* The patient is elated and abnormally euphoric but may also be irritable and rude. Intermingled with the manic or hypomanic affective changes there may be short episodes of depression.

5. *Thought and talk.* Thinking, like the general level of activity, is speeded up. Consequently, the patient may demonstrate a *flight of ideas*, the thoughts coming out in rapid succession with little connection. Thinking may also become *grandiose*, leading to *delusions* which may involve Royalty, Parliament, big business transactions, or have a religious colouring. The patient's speech may be laden with puns and wise-cracks, and these occur on the basis of '*clang associations*'.

6. *Attention.* This is short-lived, and the patient is very distractible, with frequent changes of course in his behaviour and speech.

7. *Appetite* for food and sex is increased.

What is the **differential diagnosis** of mania?

Mental disturbances which may appear to be similar to mania or hypomania include those associated with overactivity or restlessness, or with an expansive mood and grandiose thinking.

1. *G.P.I.* ('General Paralysis of the Insane' or Dementia Paralytica)

Blood and cerebrospinal fluid examination are diagnostic in this condition, which is usually associated with neurological signs and evidence of intellectual deterioration.

2. *Catatonic excitement*

The previous history and the history of the present illness are the main clues. Schizophrenic thought disorder may be in evidence, and in addition hallucinations. The latter are rare in mania.

3. *Epilepsy*

Temporal lobe epilepsy may produce states of excitement, and epilepsy of long-standing, especially if poorly controlled, can lead to psychoses in which the patient is grandiose or paranoid. The EEG may be helpful in the diagnosis.

4. *Toxic psychosis or confusional state*

Amphetamines frequently give rise to a toxic state which may resemble mania. In these states there may be clouding of consciousness, and the history and examination of the patient should lead to the exact diagnosis.

5. *Acute dissociative (hysterical) state*

This state usually follows some marked stress, and may simulate mania when occurring in the subnormal or in certain cultural groups who have not incorporated the relative stolidity of the British character.

Summarise the **treatment** of mania

1. *Drugs*

(*a*) Butyrophenones, e.g. haloperidol, are major tranquillisers, with considerable success in the treatment of mania and hypomania. In the very restless patient, the drug can be given by injection, e.g. 2·5 mg. six-hourly. When the patient becomes more co-operative and less hyperactive, haloperidol can be given orally, in a dosage of 1·5 mg. to 3 mg. three or four times daily. The drug dosage is gradually reduced to a maintenance dose.

An anti-Parkinsonian drug is prescribed in addition to the

butyrophenones, on account of the tendency to drug-induced Parkinsonian and other extrapyramidal side-effects.

(b) The phenothiazines (also major tranquillisers) are also used in treatment. Chlorpromazine is a useful phenothiazine in the management of the restless or excited patient, but large doses may be required, e.g. 400 to 1000 mg. daily, in the treatment of mania.

(c) In recent years lithium salts, in particular lithium carbonate, have been used in the treatment of mania but more commonly in an attempt to reduce the frequency of manic-depressive episodes in vulnerable patients. Lithium carbonate (250 mg. or 300 mg. capsules) is administered initially two or three times per day, the aim being to achieve a serum lithium level of between 0·6 and 1·6 meq./l. The patient is then kept on a maintenance dose, which varies from individual to individual. A long-acting preparation (Priadel) is now available, to allow less frequent drug administration. Lithium salts are slowly excreted and toxic effects are often pronounced. The most frequent features of toxicity include diarrhoea, tremor, ataxia, dizziness, thirst, polyuria and blurred vision. If the serum level reaches 3-4 meq./l. then confusion, epileptic fits, nystagmus, muscle fasciculation and vomiting may develop. Such is the nature of individual variation in response to the drug that toxicity may ensue at lower serum levels.

Contraindications to lithium therapy: renal disease, heart disease, Addison's disease and other conditions associated with faulty water and sodium metabolism.

For more details on the action and toxic effects of lithium see Section 3.

2. *ECT*

Although ECT is indicated mainly in severe psychotic depression, it is often used in the treatment of mania, as an adjunct to therapy with one of the major tranquillisers. When ECT is given in addition to one of these drugs, a severe attack of mania is likely to be terminated in the shortest possible time.

3. *Follow-up*

This is important, since mania is likely to recur or give way to depression. Once control has been established it should be maintained for at least three months.

SCHIZOPHRENIA

What is schizophrenia?

The term 'schizophrenia' is applied to psychotic reactions which usually begin in adolescence or a little later and in which occur thought disorders and emotional and behavioural disturbances; there is a tendency to withdraw from reality and to regress to a deteriorated level of conduct, frequently with hallucinations and delusions. These abnormalities occur in various combinations and mixtures, but few schizophrenic patients will exhibit all schizophrenic features. The condition may also manifest as a gradual, insidious deterioration of personality, without any florid features.

Which are the commoner schizophrenic symptoms and signs?

1. *Behaviour and drive*

Withdrawal is frequent and the term *autism* refers to a turning away from reality, with a consequent preoccupation with a phantasy world. The preoccupation with the self ('narcissism') may produce a focusing of interest on bodily health, leading to hypochondriasis or ideas about parts of the body changing. In the early stages of the illness the patient might feel unable to put his ideas into action and complain of slowness or general lack of efficiency. He may attribute his feelings of strangeness or of unreality ('depersonalisation') to outside influences, and begin to feel that his body or mind is under control ('passivity' feelings). A general lack of drive and interest is a frequent finding, especially in the chronic schizophrenic.

2. *Thought disorder*

The patient may present with complaints of muddled thoughts or of confused thinking. When thought disorder becomes fully established, *thought blocking* may be observed, i.e. the stream of thought is suddenly interrupted, and the patient may complain of crowding of his thoughts or of their being mixed up. Other manifestations of schizophrenic thought disorder include 'Knight's move' thinking, where the patient's thinking shows a devious or indirect approach as the Knight's move in chess. This and other examples of the schizophrenic's difficulty in manoeuvring associations or links in his thoughts and in thinking in *abstract concepts*, lead to incoherence of speech. The latter may become a '*word salad*' often with new words formed ('*neologisms*') and give the semblance to the observer of complete gibberish.

3. *Affect*

In the early stages of a schizophrenic illness, *depression* is commonly a feature, and may be the patient's reaction to early sinister symptoms. Inappropriate mood or *incongruity of affect* frequently supervenes, especially in the young schizophrenic. Occasionally the patient is elated or euphoric, and such a patient might show grandiose ideas or delusions. *Lability of mood* with frequent alterations in emotional display unrelated to circumstances, may occur.

Anxiety may manifest itself in the early stages of schizophrenia, usually being in the nature of the patient's attempt to erect a neurotic defence. Other neurotic features, such as phobias, obsessional features and hypochondriasis, may occur on a similar basis.

In the later stages of the illness, the commonest affective disturbance is a blunting or flattening of all emotional responses.

4. *Catatonic features*

These include:

(a) Extreme reduction of activity (*stupor*) or extreme over-activity (restlessness or *catatonic* excitement).

(b) Reactions to suggestions—either *negativism*, which implies resistance to suggestion, culminating in undue stubbornness or complete refusal to move or eat, etc.: or *automatic obedience*, whereby the patient allows his limbs or body to be placed in any position, and does not spontaneously revert to the resting pose, this is called *flexibilitas cerea* or waxy flexibility. Other features of automatic obedience include the patient's repetition of what is said to him (*echolalia*) or mimicry of the observer's actions (*echopraxia*).

(*c*) Stereotyped behaviour or postures. These refer to various facial grimacings, bodily mannerisms, aimless repetitive movements and bizarre body postures.

5. *Delusions*

Primary delusions are seen mainly in early cases of schizophrenia, and are often not discernible in the later stages because secondary delusions become elaborated on them. The primary delusion, often referred to as an *autochthonous idea*, occurs suddenly 'out of the blue', and the patient at once believes it with great conviction.

Most delusions are secondary, and are the psychotic's way of rationalising or explaining to himself his ideas or the changes which he feels in himself or in his environment. In the schizophrenic, most secondary delusions are *paranoid*, and in particular *persecutory* in nature. He may believe that the neighbours or some organisation are plotting against him.

Ideas of reference may be held, e.g. the patient sees strangers conversing and misinterprets, believing that they are talking about him. *Grandiose* delusions are sometimes seen in schizophrenia, the patient believing that he is a deity, or has royal blood or supernatural powers. *Hypochondriacal* delusions result when the patient's hypochondriacal ideas assume delusional intensity. Passivity feelings may lead the patient to believe that he is under the control of a particular object or organisation, i.e. *delusions of influence and control*.

6. *Hallucinations*

These are commonly *auditory*, the schizophrenic hearing voices which comment on his thoughts, make remarks about him, or give him messages. *Visual* hallucinations in the form of visions sometimes occur, although this type of hallucination is more characteristic of an organic state. *Tactile* or *haptic* hallucinations, e.g. of the body or parts of it being touched or interfered with, and *olfactory* hallucinations (of smell) occasionally present in schizophrenia.

7. *Personality deterioration*

Some schizophrenics do not present any of the above more florid symptoms or signs, or do so only periodically; but they may show an insidious deterioration of personality, with repercussions in their work, family and social relationships.

What **forms of schizophrenia** *occur?*

1. *Hebephrenic*

This is the classical, florid type of illness occurring in an adolescent or young adult. There is evidence of affective and thought disturbance, and frequently hallucinations and delusions. Disturbance of behaviour and volition is almost invariable. Incongruous giggling or crying is especially common.

2. *Simple*

In this form, although some of the more striking abnormalities such as hallucinations and thought disorder may occur, the illness often manifests as a gradual deterioration of personality, with changes in the affect, e.g. the young adult may become callous and unsympathetic. Drive is frequently reduced, with consequent drop in occupational efficiency. These patients may become chronically unemployed, lead the life of a vagrant, or resort to drugs or petty crime.

3. *Catatonic*

This type is characterised by catatonic features (see above), although there may well be thought disorder and hallucinations in addition. Pure catatonic states are rare.

4. *Paranoid*

Paranoid delusions of persecutory type and auditory hallucinations are the cardinal features of paranoid schizophrenia. Average age of onset is 35 years, which is later than that associated with other forms of schizophrenia; consequently there tends to be better personality and affective preservation in this form.

Paraphrenia refers to the late onset of an illness indistinguishable from paranoid schizophrenia.

5. *Schizo-affective*

This form exhibits both schizophrenic and affective (usually depressive) features, with equal prominence. Onset is usually more acute than in other forms and precipitating factors are frequently present, being of a similar nature to those elicited in depressed patients. Personality preservation tends to be good.

6. *Pseudo-neurotic*

In this type the early and neurotic defences predominate, the patient not having succumbed completely to a psychotic state. Hence obsessional and hypochondriacal features are usually present in the setting of anxiety, without any hallucinations or delusions. Although these patients do not exhibit any florid psychotic features, they are incapacitated and do not function as well as a neurotic with similar symptoms. This type of schizophrenia is often referred to as '*latent*'.

Many cases of schizophrenia do not easily lend themselves to classification in water-tight compartments. Mixed forms in fact occur with much greater frequency than pure-culture forms. Any classification is, in our present state of knowledge, mainly descriptive.

Discuss the **aetiology** of *schizophrenia*

1. *Social*

Schizophrenia is alleged to concentrate in the lowest social classes and it was originally believed that poor environmental conditions acted as causal factors in the illness. This is now explained by the 'downward drift' hypothesis, i.e. the schizophrenic, because of his illness, becomes less efficient, takes more menial employment, and may drift socially on account of alienation from his family and friends. The prevalence of schizophrenia in Europe is said to be approximately 0·85 per cent, but estimates are elusive. In various countries immigrant groups have a higher incidence than the host population.

2. *Genetic*

Genetic factors probably play some part in the aetiology of certain cases. Concordance rates which have been observed in monozygotic twins vary from nil to 86 per cent, the average figure being somewhere between 20 and 40 per cent. Approximately one-sixth of the offspring of schizophrenics develop the illness. Current evidence indicates that hereditary factors are less important in the aetiology of schizophrenia than was previously accepted and terms like 'polygenic heredity' have little credence with serious workers in the field.

3. *Personality and constitution*

It has often been believed, following the work of Kretschmer, that a particular type of body build predisposed to a schizophrenic breakdown. Supportive evidence for this hypothesis is lacking. Similarly the *schizoid* type of personality is often regarded as vulnerable, with regard to the development of schizophrenia. However, the schizoid type is found not only among those who develop the disorder, but in patients suffering from other forms of mental illness, and in people with no psychiatric morbidity. In fact, only 50 per cent of schizophrenics have a schizoid premorbid personality. If personality factors are important in vulnerability to schizophrenia, then it is not any particular type of personality, but the general mode of early personality development and parental influences on the latter that may be relevant.

4. *Family studies*

In patients with severe forms of schizophrenia, abnormal family relationships are frequently found, with the lack of an affectionate and secure environment which is necessary for the healthy development of an individual's personality. The mother (often referred to as *'schizophrenogenic'*) tends to be well-intentioned, but overprotective, ineffective and smothering; the father tends to be the less dominant parent and is either a background figure in the home, or overtly hostile to the young patient. These parents tend to deny that their offspring are ill, even if an overt psychosis is apparent. It has been suggested that schizophrenic behaviour is learned in the family through contradictory experiences— so-called *'double-bind'* communication.

5. *Metabolic*

(*a*) The hallucinogenic drug mescalin is closely related, in chemical structure, to dopamine and adrenaline. It has been postulated that in schizophrenia an abnormal metabolite, similar in action to mescalin, is developed through a faulty mechanism in the dopamine-adrenaline pathway; and that this substance acts on the brain, producing a toxic type of psychosis, presenting with the clinical features of schizophrenia. The earliest theory along these lines was the 'adrenochrome theory'. The link between catecholamines and some of the hallucinogenic compounds could be completed by the process of methylation. One of the functions of methionine is that of a methyl donor; it has been shown that administering large amounts of methionine to schizophrenics produces clinical deterioration. It is also suggested that an anti-metabolite of methionine, viz. methionine sulphoximine induces a toxic psychosis in normal people, but has no effect on schizophrenics.

(b) Numerous investigations have taken place to demonstrate the presence, in the blood of schizophrenic patients, of a toxic substance. It has been variously found that plasma taken from schizophrenics disturbs the carbohydrate metabolism of chicken red blood corpuscles and other experimental preparations.

(c) Possible role of serotonin (5-hydroxytryptamine). Since it was shown that serotonin is an antagonist of the psychotomimetic drug LSD, efforts have been made to implicate serotonin in biochemical theories of schizophrenia. There is slight evidence that tryptamine excretion is increased during clinical exacerbations in schizophrenic patients.

(d) The chemical resemblance of melatonin to the hallucinogenic drug harmine has been remarked upon; and it has been noted recently that melanin is deposited in excessive amounts in some tissues of schizophrenic patients, especially those taking chlorpromazine. In humans, pigmentation is normally decreased by melatonin; the theory is that that in schizophrenia the normal route of synthesis of melatonin from serotonin is blocked, so that instead of melatonin hallucinogenic compounds like harmine are produced.

(e) *Gjessing's syndrome.* This refers to a rare form of schizophrenia, viz. periodic catatonia, in which variations in nitrogen retention are found to be associated with changes in mental state. This type of metabolic abnormality has not been confirmed in the great majority of schizophrenics.

6. *Neurological and neurophysiological*

Although the brains of schizophrenics do not exhibit any abnormalities which are not attributable to artefact, there are suggestions that brain function may be disturbed in certain cases of schizophrenia. For instance, there is a higher incidence of abnormal EEGs than in the general population but they are not specific for schizophrenia and vary from epileptic to immature records. Other neurophysiological investigations point to altered states of arousal in schizophrenics, inferring functional changes in the nervous system.

There is also evidence that disorder of the temporal lobes of the brain may lead to schizophrenic-like psychoses as in certain temporal lobe epileptics. A direct causal relationship is still unproven though some implicate the role of anti-epileptic drugs in producing mental illness in chronic epileptics. Certain anti-convulsant drugs can interfere with vitamin B_{12} and folate metabolism and deficiency of these factors can provoke various types of neuro-psychiatric sequelae.

In summary, schizophrenia probably consists of a variety of similar syndromes. The aetiology is most likely multifactorial, and the parts played by heredity, biochemistry, family constellation, etc., must vary considerably from patient to patient. Presumably the balance between vulnerability and environmental stress will in many cases determine whether the illness becomes clinically manifest. In some, where the genetic loading is high (possibly with consequent related metabolic abnormality) the patient may become mentally ill irrespective of environmental influences. In others, marked psychological stress may be necessary to precipitate the psychosis. Adolf Meyer coined the concept of the '*schizophrenic reaction-type*' which underlined the fact that schizophrenia is often not merely an irrevocable disease process, but the reaction of an individual whose vulnerability is biologically determined but whose illness is finally precipitated by psychological stress.

Discuss the **prognosis** of schizophrenia

With modern treatment there is an approximately 70 per cent chance of a schizophrenic with a first breakdown leading a normal life for at least two years after the illness and 50 per cent chance after five years. Only 30 per cent will be completely free of all clinical features; but social and occupational adjustments are the most important indices of ability to live a normal life in the community.

The prognosis of a schizophrenic illness depends on several variables:

1. *The nature of the illness.* The more severe forms of schizophrenia, e.g. with strong constitutional loading, an insidious course and with subsequent personality deterioration, are often designated 'process schizophrenia' or 'nuclear type' schizophrenia. These constitute the hard-core problems and carry a worse prognosis than the so-called 'schizophrenic reactions' or 'schizophreniform psychoses', which are more short-lived and tend not to lead to any deterioration of the personality.

2. Strong hereditary loading or classical schizophrenogenic family.constellation tend to carry poor prognosis.

3. If *precipitating factors* are present as in a schizophrenic reaction, and can be remedied or are unlikely to be repeated, the prognosis is improved.

4. Acuteness of *onset* carries a far better prognosis than an insidious one.

5. The presence of an affective admixture such as a depressive element is a good feature.

6. *Treatment.* Adequate treatment, and rehabilitation if necessary, prior to discharge from hospital, and suitable follow-up in the community with continuation of medication are factors likely to promote a satisfactory outcome.

7. *Reduction of environmental stress.* If a patient after hospital treatment returns to an abnormal family constellation with an emotionally charged atmosphere, the remission of his illness may be short-lived. Similarly, stress, speed or responsibility at work may militate against the patient's continued well-being.

How is schizophrenia treated?

1. *Environmental factors.* If there are any environmental stresses operating to the detriment of the patient's health, an attempt should be made to reduce their impact. This may

mean dealing with personal, school or work situations, or more likely with family tensions. The family of a schizophrenic is often taken into the treatment situation and counselled by doctor or social worker. The patient may be encouraged to leave home and live more independently, e.g. in hostel or suitable lodgings. The patient and his family may be dealt with in selected hospital units as a disturbed family complex, the patient being considered as only one manifestation of a sick family. This approach, pioneered in this country by Laing, attempts to employ some of the principles of existentialism in a rather esoteric form of psychotherapy. The treatment process tends to be lengthy and time-consuming for the patient, his family and the doctor and results to date have not justified the publicity it has received.

2. *Drugs.* Phenothiazines are the drugs of choice. Chlorpromazine is more useful in the restless or hyperactive patient, whereas the piperazine group of phenothiazines, e.g. trifluoperazine, are indicated for the withdrawn anergic type of patient. The dosage of these drugs varies enormously and depends on the needs of the patient and the occurrence of side-effects. In an acute schizophrenic illness, the necessary dosage of chlorpromazine is unlikely to be less than 100 mg. thrice daily. These drugs are available as tablets, syrup, or injections; long-term medication with phenothiazines is indicated in most cases of schizophrenia and may be given as tablets (most phenothiazines), long-acting capsules (e.g. trifluoperazine), or longer-acting injections (e.g. fluphenazine). Two preparations of the latter are available, viz. enanthate and decanoate. These drugs are initially given in a test dose of 12·5 mg. which is followed about 10 days later by a full 25 mg. injection. In some patients, phenothiazine maintenance requirements can be provided by a single injection of one of these drugs every 2, 3, or 4 weeks, depending on individual needs. The main indications for these 'depot' doses are for chronic schizophrenics who relapse when they stop taking their tablets, and for those who have a general reluctance to take any drugs which are prescribed for them.

In patients who do not respond satisfactorily to phenothiazine drugs, there are three non-phenothiazine alternative groups of drugs. Butyrophenones, e.g. haloperidol and triperidol, have a similar type of action, and are useful where behavioural problems persist and with phenothiazine-resistant psychotic symptoms.

Diphenylbutylpiperidines, e.g. pimozide, although virtually ineffective on their own, can be given in combination with phenothiazines, and a long-acting preparation is now available. Thioxanthenes are the third group and there is a long-acting form: flupenthixol.

3. *ECT*. There is a limited usefulness of electroplexy in the treatment of schizophrenia, viz.:

(a) catatonic states, e.g. stupor;
(b) where a depressive component is marked;
(c) often recommended in an acute schizophrenic illness (in addition to drugs), especially if it is the first breakdown in a young person; there is evidence that ECT helps to cut short the attack.

4. *Rehabilitation*. This is indicated especially in the patient who has suffered several schizophrenic breakdowns and/or has evidence of personality deterioration. Rehabilitation programmes (for psychiatric in-patients or day hospital patients) include emphasis on improving the occupational and social levels of functioning of the patient. Industrial therapy, involving some approximation to a factory atmosphere, often with incentives, is a useful adjunct in rehabilitation. Behavioural techniques, e.g. token economy programmes, are sometimes employed to rectify faulty habits or modes of behaviour.

5. *Supportive psychotherapy* is often helpful. In the U.K. it is usual to offer superficial support in addition to drugs, but in the U.S.A. intensive psychotherapy is often practised.

Hospital in-patient treatment, as opposed to out-patient treatment, is indicated:

(a) in the first schizophrenic breakdown;
(b) if there is a marked disturbance of behaviour, or the patient is a danger to himself or to others;
(c) where there are unsurmountable stresses in the environment which are thought to militate against the patient's recovery.

What are **paranoid states** *or paranoid psychoses?*

The term 'paranoid' is usually applied to major mental illnesses in which the prominent symptoms are persistent delusions of a persecutory or grandiose nature. In the past, *'paranoia'* and other paranoid states were often categorised on the basis of preservation of personality, presence or absence of hallucinations, and the degree to which the delusions were 'systematised'.

Paranoid symptoms may occur in a variety of conditions, and where the paranoid features include delusions, the term 'paranoid psychosis' is applicable. Paranoid states or psychoses are not disease entities, but may occur on the basis of any of the following mental illnesses:

1. *Paranoid schizophrenia* and *paraphrenia.* Paranoid delusions and auditory hallucinations are usually present.

2. *Psychotic depression.* The patient with a deep depression may feel guilty and unworthy and project these ideas about himself on to others, resulting in persecutory ideas or delusions.

3. *Organic states.* The patient with delirium misinterprets his surroundings, is in a state of intense fear, and often develops ideas or delusions of persecution. Similarly, the dementing patient who is very forgetful and loses things, projects his disability on to the actions of others and accuses them of stealing from him.

4. Drug-induced, e.g. through the action of amphetamine.

5. Long-standing *epileptics* (especially of temporal lobe type) occasionally develop paranoid psychoses.

6. *Paranoid reaction.* It is possible for someone to develop a paranoid state as a reaction to some stress. In such a case, there is often a constitutional predisposition to react in this way, but when delusions develop the condition may be indistinguishable from paranoid schizophrenia. Some of these cases were often labelled 'paranoia' in the past.

7. *Paranoid personality.* This is a personality disorder, which occasionally spills over into a paranoid reaction, following psychological or environmental stress. There are two types of paranoid personality:

   (*a*) sensitive and suspicious;
   (*b*) individuals who cling to some belief or cause tenaciously, often having *'overvalued ideas'* which do not amount to

delusions. These people are frequently 'anti-this' or 'anti-that' and go through life with a very large chip on their shoulder.

The mental mechanism concerned in paranoid states is *projection*, and any delusions that arise follow misinterpretations based on this mechanism. Early studies of the psychopathology of paranoid states including Freud's classical account of the Schreber case confirmed that the psychological conflicts in a paranoid patient are of a homosexual nature. As a corollary, it is well known that homosexuals are prone to develop paranoid states.

PSYCHONEUROSES

What is meant by the **psychoneuroses?**

These are illnesses which comprise a group of non-organic mental disorders which though particularly distressing to the patient, do not possess the qualities of severe affective change or thought disturbance which are associated with the psychoses. This definition, in other words, says that psychoneuroses are not psychoses, and we next have to differentiate between the neuroses and the psychoses.

Freud regarded the neuroses as the result of conflict between the ego and the id, and the psychoses as an analogous outcome of a similar disturbance in the relation between the ego and its environment (outer world). In the neuroses the influence of reality is decisive, but in the psychoses it is the id which takes over and a loss of reality must be an inherent element. A more succinct definition from Freud's point of view is 'neurosis does not deny the existence of reality, it merely tries to ignore it; psychosis denies it and tries to substitute something else for it'. Many consider there is no real distinction between a neurosis and a psychosis; what was at one time considered to be neurotic is now recognised as being an early stage of a psychosis, such as in pseudo-neurotic schizophrenia, and some psychopathic problems.

A constitutional neurotic type as indicating genetic determinants for neurotic illness has been postulated, with the corollary that there are also genetic determinants for psychotic illness, but conclusive evidence for this has not been forthcoming.

Classify the **psychoneuroses**

These generally constitute six reactions: (1) Anxiety, (2) Dissociative, (3) Conversion, (4) Phobic, (5) Obsessive compulsive, and (6) Depressive. It should be noted that these are reactions and not diseases and that one reaction does not exclude another;

in fact, several can co-exist, though many disorders are pre-dominantly of one type.

Discuss the **anxiety reactions**

Anxiety need not be evidence of mental disease for it may serve a useful purpose. On difficult occasions, the normal person exhibits anxiety, such as during examinations or when failure may threaten the existence or self-esteem of the individual. Anxiety, therefore, has a special significance for the conquest of the environment or for self-realisation and a culture which excites this pattern of behaviour is more likely to achieve success in these fields than one which does not. Achievement in physical and mental activity and risk-taking activities such as exploration, mountaineering, sailing and gambling may cancel out anxiety and may even be of prophylactic value. 'Courage, in the final analysis, is nothing but an affirmative answer to the shocks of existence, which must be borne for the actualisation of one's own nature'.

Cannon, whose physiological studies on fear and rage defined the biological aspects of anxiety, contributed further and showed that anxiety should be seen as an expression of interference with homeostatic equilibrium which could be threatened, broken down or could try to re-establish itself at a different level.

Other physiological aspects

Grinker induced stress experimentally in volunteers, measured the physiological response including serum and urinary cortisol and studied the specificity of the various stress situations.

Funkenstein studied the cardiovascular aspects of emotional responses of students to acute emergency. He defined two categories, those who reacted with 'anger out' and showed cardiovascular responses similar to those produced by noradrenaline, while those who reacted with 'anger in' or severe anxiety had a response similar to that produced by adrenaline. Neurosurgeons have shown that ablation of certain parts of the cortex may result in absence of anxiety. The exact aetiology is unknown but a number of theories have emerged including genetic, biochemical and neurophysiological.

Kelly measured forearm blood flow as an index of anxiety.

With the patient reclining comfortably, recordings are made of forearm blood flow, heart rate and blood pressure during 'basal' (resting) conditions for 15 minutes. Anxiety is then introduced by asking the subject to perform difficult arithmetic as quickly as possible. He is also continually harassed and criticised while a metronome is beating at a two-second rate.

The differences between 'basal' and 'stress' measurements are calculated as percentage increases and this is regarded as a reliable estimate of physiological reactivity or lability. 'Basal' forearm blood flow is considered to be an approximate measurement of *free-floating* anxiety, whereas 'stress' values measure *situational* anxiety.

Sodium lactate infusions have also been used to provoke a 'stress' reaction.

Cultural factors

These are probably significant, for in a society where anxiety is fostered, a number will over-react or fail to master the environment and be subject to disability. While, theoretically, infantile experience should be paramount, anxiety can be grafted on in adult life to cultural groups who had previously not shown such reactions.

The specific event

This is frequently volunteered by the patient as the cause of his initial anxiety attack. Accidents and operations are frequently quoted, with frights, separations, sudden privations, births of siblings and sudden environmental changes being less commonly mentioned.

Describe the symptomatology of anxiety attacks

These are usually acute or chronic.

Acute

The picture is that of over-stimulation of the autonomic nervous system. The heart rate is accelerated and the apex beat is more forcible with, in some instances, praecordial discomfort or pain. Respiration rate is increased and the consequent hyperventilation produces its own syndrome. Dyspnoea, dysphagia and a feeling of choking are common and on occasions there is respiratory distress. Urgency of micturition, diarrhoea, weakness of the knees or a total feeling of exhaustion can occur. Pupils dilate, sweating may be extreme, the mouth is dry, the hands tremble, the facial appearance is over-anxious.

Chronic

This is really a persistence of the acute attack in attenuated form, liable to periodic exacerbations. It may be associated with 'startle' reactions which are triggered off by some sudden shock. In servicemen this could be a car back-firing or some other loud noise like an aircraft swooping overhead. The facies is constantly anxious, there is a marked tremor and sweating of the hands, tachycardia and disturbed sleep, the patient being frequently wakened by terrifying dreams. There is a general lowering of efficiency with impaired concentration and a tendency to hypochondriasis.

What is meant by 'fixated' anxiety?

This is said to occur when the patient focuses his symptoms on an organ or region of the body, and is attributed to the concomitant physiological disturbance such as tachycardia, dysphagia or praecordial pain with palpitations. He is usually seen first by physicians for suspected peptic ulcer, bowel disorders, heart disease, thyrotoxicosis and hyperinsulinism.

These symptoms do not occur in isolation but are usually associated with a large range of psychiatric disturbances. It is therefore important to make, not only a qualitative diagnosis but a quantitative one, in order to decide how big a part it plays in the total psychiatric reaction.

Discuss the differential diagnosis of anxiety

In the chronic state, this is mainly confined to the exclusion of thyrotoxicosis which is now more easily defined with laboratory tests. Even the acute attack can be mistaken for thyrotoxicosis and the two conditions cannot be differentiated by the presence of an immediate psychological precipitant, for this could be common to both. Rigid exclusion of the thyrotoxicosis is essential.

G

Other organic states which are mistaken for anxiety are lesions in the region of the diencephalon, carotid sinus hypersensitivity, heart disease and addiction to dextroamphetamine sulphate. Some organic cerebral states may heighten the anxiety features because of intellectual deficit.

Discuss the **treatment of anxiety states**

The acute attack. If severe, this may require very heavy sedation, if not continuous narcosis. A useful compromise is amylobarbitone sodium 200 mg. three times a day, though this should not be maintained for more than two or three days and preferably under reliable supervision because of the danger of addiction. Patient's remedies, such as alcohol and other agents may have to be withdrawn.

Specific remedies

Anxiolytic drugs. Many of these are now being marketed, the most popular being diazepam (Valium) and chlordiazepoxide (Librium). All investigations to date have shown that these anxiolytic agents when given orally are no more effective than placebos and do not match up to amylobarbitone sodium. Nevertheless, some patients do claim that they get relief from their anxiety with the administration of these drugs and their continued prescription is likely. As it is increasingly realised that anxiety can co-exist with other psychiatric conditions, particularly depression, mild anti-depressants of the dibenzepin group have been used and in controlled trials these have been shown to be more effective than diazepam and chlordiazepoxide.

Hospital treatment

This should be reserved for severe cases only, but as many of the less severe are adulterated with drug addiction or alcoholism admission to hospital will be necessary for them too.

Abreaction techniques

Narco-analysis. This is an exploratory method using an intravenous narcotic such as sodium thiopentone 0·5 g., dissolved in 20 ml. of distilled water. It is given intravenously and injected slowly. In the pre-narcotic stage the patient may be less inhibited and be able to discuss and recall events which he had previously repressed.

Narcosynthesis. The treatment is similar to narco-analysis, but the patient is encouraged to re-experience the intense emotion accompanying the event which precipitated the attack of anxiety and thus deal with it more adequately. In practice narcosynthesis and narco-analysis are not discrete treatments, but are usually combined.

Ether abreaction. Ether is given with an open mask and in the pre-narcotic state the patient may become excitable and re-live previous experiences with a resultant reduction in tension. Seldom used.

Carbon dioxide therapy which consists of a mixture of 30 per cent carbon dioxide and 70 per cent oxygen. This is breathed through a mask for 30 to 40 inhalations, after which the patient enters a subconscious stage and becomes excited with the accompaniment of violent muscular movements and a concomitant abreaction. Seldom used.

Methedrine. Ten to 20 mg. are usually combined with 0·5 g. of sodium thiopentone. This is given intravenously and the patient may become extremely talkative and be more communicative than he normally would be, with resultant uncovering of aggravating and precipitating factors. With this treatment there is a real danger of addiction to both methedrine and barbiturates and the former is no longer available for prescription by general practitioners.

Continuous narcosis

The purpose is to maintain the patient asleep for long periods, the objective being 20 hours sleep in 24 hours, though this is not easy to maintain. Amylobarbitone sodium 200 mg. doses six-hourly is given, and it can be potentiated with chlorpromazine 50 mg. three times a day. The patient is kept in a darkened and quiet room and all his needs, including feeding and toilet, are catered for. Fluid intake and output are carefully controlled, the urine examined repeatedly for ketones, and the patient strictly supervised in order to make sure that he does not suffocate himself by turning his face into his pillow. The blood pressure should be monitored. A special pillow through which the patient can breathe is essential. Some now recommend this treatment for the weaning of severe forms of drug addiction.

Diazepam. Twenty milligrams is given intravenously as in anaesthesia. It has an interesting action in that it does not produce loss of consciousness but the patient has an amnesia for the injection, feels very relaxed and is ready to go home shortly afterwards. It is being increasingly used on out-patients, particularly where phobic features are in evidence. It is still too early to evaluate its usefulness, though, as one would expect, early results are encouraging.

Psychotherapy. See Section 18.

Group therapy. See Section 18.

Describe the **main features of phobic anxiety**

This is a form of anxiety where the phobia acts as a defence, often an inadequate one, to protect the patient from situations and circumstances which may predispose to or initiate the anxiety attacks. The patient recognises that his fear is irrational but is unable to overcome it and is usually unaware of its unconscious origin.

Symptomatology

This may be protean and extend beyond the declaration of the patient's specific or general phobia. It may be heavily adulterated with the symptoms of acute anxiety attacks which in turn may excite the *hyperventilation syndrome* and even produce transient loss or disturbance of consciousness. In such cases depersonalisation is common and the condition may be mistaken for a temporal lobe attack. Situations which are feared are, in the male, sitting in the barber's chair, and in the female, leaving home unescorted, travelling on buses or doing shopping. Both sexes are frequently affected by their inability to enter into situations where there are crowds of people and where they are unable to escape because of a closed door, such as a church service or a concert. The condition can be very crippling and many patients are unable to get to work or lead an ordinary life, and a number resort to alcohol and drugs in order to give themselves the confidence they lack.

Discuss the treatment of phobic anxiety

A variety of measures have been used including intravenous barbiturates, psychotherapy and behaviour therapy. Recently intravenous acetylcholine has been gaining a reputation as a useful measure in de-conditioning the patient. For fuller details see Section 18.

What is hysteria?

Hysterical, or dissociative or conversion reactions, are common psychiatric disorders which occur in a variety of situations and have a variety of meanings. They can assume protean forms including amnesias, tremors, anaesthesias, paralyses of limbs, hyperventilation attacks, mutism, deafness, blindness, somnambulism or attacks resembling those of epilepsy. Two major clinical groups are defined: (1) the hysterical character, and (2) hysterical symptoms.

Describe the hysterical character

These patients are usually female, and they are flamboyantly sexual with a display of coquetry, and in the rare cases in men there is usually effeminacy. Such an attitude usually projects the individual into situations where the apparent sexual goal is within reach and then, as a defence, gross hysterical behaviour becomes mobilised. They are unpredictable, over-suggestible, over-imaginative and insincere, with a compulsive love-hunger, high dependency needs for approval, a dramatic sense and exhibit sharp reactions to disappointment. They tend to confuse phantasy with reality and are prone to a variety of somatic complaints as well as to hysterical ones, such as skin reactions. The apparent exuberance they display conceals a shallow affectivity, and the scenes and disturbances with which they frequently surround themselves are evidence of reality testing. They may be responsible for unwarranted claims against doctors, for the need for publicity drives them to litigation. They are very disturbed persons, and their condition, though apparently neurotic, is very close to a malignant psychotic state. Individual psychotherapy would appear to be the most hopeful form of treatment, but even then the outlook should be guarded. Most are, like the psychopath, immature, and maturation may take place slowly.

Discuss hysterical symptoms

Psychopathology. This is basically a dissociative mechanism which is a reaction to an anxiety-producing situation. As a result of the dissociation the underlying anxiety is *converted* to a variety of signs and symptoms giving rise to the term *hysterical conversion reaction.* Some doubt the unconscious nature of these hysterical symptoms and Szasz stresses that the hysterical symptomatology is a form of language used by the individual to convey his distress and secure from society that which he requires to relieve it. With hysteria, therefore, we permit oblique references to problems where direct statements would not be countenanced and it is therefore a form of 'hinting', that is dropping clues to those who claim they are experienced in recognising them.

It is equivalent to a distress signal flown from a ship's mast, but it does not necessarily convey to the observer the nature of the distress. It can mean that there is fire, plague or mutiny aboard or that the ship is sinking. It may not indicate anything more grave than that the ship's captain has forgotten to post his football coupon, but the triviality of the problem may not modify the urgency of the signal. In many instances there is an inverse relationship.

The commoner symptoms are amnesia, multiple personality, somnambulism or sleep-walking, the Ganser-like syndrome, hysterical convulsions, paralyses, tremors and spasms, sensory disturbances, pain, symptoms such as blindness and blepharospasm, dysphagia, respiratory tics and nocturnal enuresis.

What is the Ganser syndrome?

This is a condition which has accumulated a variety of names such as 'prison psychosis' because of its frequent occurrence among prisoners, the syndrome of approximate answers, and hysterical pseudodementia. Ganser's original syndrome dealt with patients who, following cerebral trauma or in the course of an acute psychosis, develop clouding of consciousness with characteristic verbal responses to questions, such as the syndrome of approximate answers, and whose illnesses terminate abruptly with a subsequent amnesia. The term 'Ganser syndrome' has been adulterated to include conditions with Ganser-like symptoms such as those described above. Differentiation between Ganser-like symptoms and frank malingering can be very difficult and in many instances the two are identical.

Discuss the **differential diagnosis of hysteria?**

Diagnosis rests on (*a*) the exclusion of the organic, (*b*) the definition of an adequate and fully relevant psychopathology, and (*c*) the removal of symptoms by dealing with the problem with the appropriate psychiatric treatment. It very rarely presents after the age of 40 and in people with a good pre-morbid record without such previous history the chances are that any symptom which may resemble an hysterical one is probably of organic origin. Neurological conditions which have not yet produced the classical signs, particularly those involving the corpus striatum may be confused with hysterical symptoms.

Suggestibility. This is an essential feature of the hysteric and Hull's Body-Sway test, which consists of the experimenter suggesting to the patient who stands with his eyes closed that he is falling forward, is frequently used. The amount of sway is measured and scored. More detailed investigations have not shown this method to be particularly reliable.

What is meant by **compensation neurosis?**

This is a condition which incorporates a number of neurotic symptoms associated with a traumatic situation, either physical or psychological, where the responsible agent is also responsible in law, and the victim, if he wins his case, is entitled to financial gain. The various groups can be divided into (1) the genuine case, (2) the sick claimant with a genuine disability but where there are doubts about the part played by the accident in producing his total disability, (3) the constitutionally unstable who is a ripe candidate for compensation neurosis and who projects his lifelong history of inadequacy on to a traumatic situation, and (4) the malingerer who may also be constitutionally unstable but who sees in the accident an honourable escape from an intolerable situation at work.

Accurate information from these patients is sometimes very difficult to obtain and they are unlikely to admit to facts in their history which would prejudice their compensation claim. On the other hand, a very careful history may still yield dependable information about the patient's pre-morbid state, even if in a negative way, for they not infrequently deny even the slightest evidence of the normal insecurities to which all men are heir. They would insist that they have an impeccable family history, a most secure home background, a complete absence of neurotic traits in childhood, a stable and most successful employment record, a happy married life and no history of illness even of a trivial nature until the accident, when catastrophe overtook them. If all this were true, then the patient should be capable of recovering from the most extreme stresses imaginable, and the relatively minor stress of the accident should hardly be noticed.

Discuss **obsessional neurosis**

It is a state in which the patient unconsciously tries to control his anxiety by means of persistent and repetitive thoughts and acts. Whenever a patient complains of some mental compulsion, so that he does not willingly entertain it but, on the contrary, does his utmost to get rid of it, that is an obsession.

Psychopathology. This is dependent on an understanding of the *anal character*. Patients tend to be orderly, parsimonious and obstinate, qualities alleged to be developed by the child during habit-training.

Ritual behaviour is a very common feature in obsessional neurosis and the superstitions of the compulsive neurosis closely resemble those found in primitive people, a fact which has been pointed out by Frazer in *The Golden Bough*.

Ceremonial and obsessive acts are partly a defence against temptation and partly a protection against the misfortune expected. Protective measures rapidly become ineffective and are replaced by prohibitions and at an even later stage the performances which were initially defensive approximate more and more to the proscribed actions they were originally designed to prevent.

Undoing. This is a feature of obsessional states which is related to reaction formation and is the adoption of an attitude that contradicts the original one. Something is done, either in fact or magically, which is the opposite of that which either in fact or in imagination has been done before. It is seen in certain obsessional symptoms which consist of two components, the second being a complete rebuttal of the first; for example, the person who first has to turn the gas tap on in order to turn it off. Expiation, which is designed to annul previous acts and represents a magical undoing, can appear paradoxical when the obsession is not to do the opposite but to repeat the same act. The aim of this obsession is to carry out the same act freed of its secret unconscious meaning, or with the opposite unconscious meaning. If some part of the original impulse insinuates itself again into the repetition, which was intended as an expiation, further repetition of the act becomes necessary.

Failure of the act of undoing may result in (1) an increase in the number of repetitions as complete reassurance is not obtained with any one performance; (2) some forms of counting compulsions, the unconscious meaning of which is to count the number of repetitions; (3) the ever-widening scope of the rituals; (4) obsessive doubts which may reflect doubt as to whether the undoing has succeeded; and (5) the futility of all these measures.

Isolation. This is another common defence mechanism of obsessional neurosis. Although the patient may not have forgotten the pathogenic traumata, he has lost trace of their associations and emotional significance. Any attempt to demonstrate these associations is resisted like the hysteric resists the reactivation of repressed memories, and a counter cathexis is operating, the function of which is to keep apart what should be connected. Because of this, repulsive ideas like murder and incest may reach consciousness as obsessions, but they are securely isolated from action, although blasphemies may be explained as a failure at isolation in that what was intended to be a religious ritual becomes debased.

The ego in obsessional neurosis is very dependent on super-ego influences and this is reflected in symptomatology. Ambivalent attitudes may be developed so that obsessional neurotics are frequently able to meet the demands of a rigid super-ego and at the same time gratify their libidinous urges as is seen classically in the compulsive masturbator, who may ring himself with a variety of rituals, yet indulge his habit to a greater degree than those who have no such obsessional defence.

The *thinking* in obsessional neurosis is very close to the magical thinking of primitive people and frequently contains archaic references.

Describe the **clinical features of obsessional neurosis**

These are usually divided into three groups: (1) obsessional thoughts, (2) obsessional acts and (3) obsessional fears.

1. Obsessional thoughts or ruminations may be associated with a whole range of subjects. The commoner ones are persistent doubting (*folie de doute*) as to whether doors are locked or gas taps are turned off. Sometimes it may be a pre-occupation with a bad word, oath or blasphemy, or with a hostile intention. Pre-occupation with depersonalisation is not uncommon, particularly in adolescent girls.

2. Obsessional acts may be excited by obsessional thoughts, but they frequently exist by themselves. They may be elaborate rituals associated with bathing or washing or in preparation for going to bed. They may, like the thoughts, have a primitive or magical component and are designed to placate an omnipotent power. Over-protection, over-solicitude, avoidance of contamination, touching, counting, persistent note-taking and recording of each and every event, no matter how trivial, are only a few of the manifestations.

3. Obsessional phobias are usually associated with anxiety, and they are frequent accompaniments of the thoughts and acts described above. Fears of dirt or contamination may lead to frequent washing and avoidance of touching certain objects or people. Some patients with fears of contaminating their loved ones will not bring outdoor shoes into the house, but will leave them outside in a dish of disinfectant. Some with fears of spreading germs will scrub their hands till they are raw and damage them further with frequent bathing in concentrated antiseptic. Fears of harming their children may lead them to undertake elaborate rituals to avoid such misfortune. Knives are locked up and the key secreted in a place which is again rendered inaccessible, perhaps by some magical incantation which makes its hiding-place taboo. Certain mannerisms in dress may be due to fears of chills or colds, and some patients disturb the office staff with whom they work by insisting that windows are kept tightly shut and they themselves wear sheets of cardboard under their jackets and look quite ridiculous in this protective garb.

4. Obsessions and psychosis. On occasions a schizophrenic psychosis may develop out of an obsessional neurosis and in this case one says that the obsessional neurosis has decompensated. The residual picture of schizophrenia is heavily adulterated with obsessional features.

Discuss the **treatment of obsessional neurosis**

This will vary in method and result, according to the purity and severity of the reaction. Because of inability to associate freely analytical therapy is unlikely to be successful, although most people do give it a trial. An adulterating depressive element will respond to anti-depressant measures and if there is decompensation into a schizophrenic illness it will require the treatment of schizophrenia. Prefrontal leucotomy has been recommended in the most severe and malignant cases, and the operation of choice today is the bilateral undercutting of areas 9 and 10. As many of the rituals are intimately associated with the patient's family, removing them from home for a period of observation in hospital is a useful measure. This permits a more accurate formulation of the problem, damps down the aggravating factors and ensures co-operation with treatment. Even a few days in hospital can, with the help of adequate tranquillisers, convert an impossible situation into one of manageable proportions.

Severe obsessional states are rarely met after the age of 55, which could be interpreted that a number of these patients do remit spontaneously; on the other hand it may be rather hazardous to leave a patient indefinitely without treatment because of the risk of suicide, or decompensation into a schizophrenic illness.

What is meant by **anankastic personality?**

This includes a combination of various character traits, such as a general feeling of insecurity with a tendency to attribute blame to oneself and to doubt one's decisions and actions. Such individuals are constantly anxious and apprehensive and readily suffer from guilt. To reassure themselves and relieve their feelings of foreboding, they indulge in repetitive checking and re-checking. The latter features are of course compulsive acts when they reach abnormal proportions. Allied to these features, anankasts also exhibit rigidity in attitude, extreme cautiousness and try to maintain perfectionist and high ethical standards. It can be seen that this personality amounts very much to an obsessional, only more so! The anankastic label is a rather outdated one, though still used by some.

In the current international classification of diseases, it is bracketed with obsessive-compulsive personality.

What is meant by neurasthenia?

This is now an outmoded term with a variety of interpretations; for example, persistent tiredness and anergia is commonly seen in depressive states, easy fatiguability with complete exhaustion in anxiety states, and the perseverative reiteration of these complaints may be part of a schizophrenic picture. Generally in the older literature it was another term for a depressive reaction but it could equally be applied to some forms of neurotic behaviour.

Discuss the depersonalisation syndrome

The four salient features are:

1. Feelings of unreality.
2. An unpleasant quality associated with these feelings.
3. The non-delusional nature of the experience.
4. The associated affective disturbance (predominantly depression).

Four aetiological categories have been defined:

1. Disturbances of a particular psychological function.
2. Cortical dysfunction either specific or secondary.
3. Psychoanalytical theories which suggest disturbances in psychological development.
4. A form of schizophrenia.

The following findings have been listed:

Positive findings. (1) Onset is practically always sudden. (2) Most typically, onset is in adolescence or early maturity. (3) It occurs as a symptom in a very wide range of psychiatric disorders. (4) It can occur in normal people as a fleeting experience, e.g. in fatigue, after anaesthesia, and experimentally during mescalin intoxication. (5) It is reversible and can recover completely and spontaneously. (6) It is significantly related to relaxation following intense or prolonged stimulation, psychological or physical. (7) It can be relieved by stimulation. (8) It can be experienced in the psychological field whether cognitive, affective or conative. (9) There is a tendency for it to occur in the more intelligent. (10) There is a tendency for it to occur in the emotionally immature. (11) There is a high incidence of unsatisfactory parent-child relationships. (12) There is a high incidence of non-specific mild abnormalities in the EEG.

Negative findings. (1) It is not a disorder of visual perception. (2) It cannot be accounted for in neurological terms by any known focal lesion. (3) There is no specific relationship with anatomical disease of the brain. (4) There is a relative absence of olfactory, gustatory, or auditory derealisation. (5) It is extremely rare in children. (6) It is practically never found in paranoia.

Differential diagnosis

It may be difficult to distinguish it from a *schizophrenic illness* in a young person, and also a *temporal lobe epilepsy*; this diagnosis is not usually made in the absence of fits and other features of the disease. The EEG can be abnormal with depersonalisation, but is usually an immature record and does not show the focal disturbance of an epileptic nature found in temporal lobe lesions.

SECTION 12

ALCOHOLISM AND DRUG ADDICTION

What is meant by **drug addiction and dependence?**

The World Health Organisation has defined drug addiction as a state of periodic or chronic intoxication, detrimental to the individual and to society, produced by the repeated consumption of a drug (natural or synthetic). Characteristics of addiction include:

1. Overpowering desire or need (compulsion) to continue taking the drug and to obtain it by any means.

2. Tendency to increase the dose.

3. Psychological and sometimes physical *dependence* on the effects of the drug.

At times, attempts have been made to distinguish between drug addiction and drug *habituation*, e.g. the latter differed from addiction in that it created a desire but not a compulsion to continue taking the drug.

In 1964, the W.H.O. recommended that '*drug dependence*' be substituted for the terms addiction or habituation. Drug dependence may either be psychological or physical, or both, and there are different types, depending on the drug involved, e.g. morphia, barbiturate, alcohol, cocaine, amphetamine, LSD and cannabis.

The second report of the Brain Committee (1965) took note of the increasing incidence of addiction to heroin and cocaine and proposed changes aimed at greater *control* of drugs. These changes, which were later embodied in the Dangerous Drugs Act (1967) included (1) a system of notification of addicts, the addict being defined as 'a person who, as a result of repeated administration, has an overpowering desire for its continuance, but who does not require it for the relief of organic disease'; (2) the setting up of special treatment centres; (3) restriction of prescriptions for heroin and cocaine to doctors attached to these treatment centres.

Describe **recent legislation on drugs**

The Misuse of Drugs Act (1971) has been the prominent landmark in new legislation in recent years. It repeals the following Acts:

The Drugs (Prevention of Misuse) Act (1964)
The Dangerous Drugs Act (1965)
The Dangerous Drugs Act (1967)

The new Act embodies many of the features of these Acts which have been repealed, e.g. system of notification of addicts, restrictions on prescriptions and on importation of drugs and penalties for unlawful possession. The Act distinguishes between unlawful possession and trafficking, increasing the penalties for the latter. It also deals with the question of irresponsible prescribing by doctors and the careful keeping of drug registers by pharmacists.

The Misuse of Drugs Act has an appended schedule of Controlled Drugs. Schedule 2 drugs include cocaine, opium, methadone, morphine, pethidine and related derivatives; also codeine, amphetamines, methaqualone, methylphenidate, phenmetrazine and related compounds. Schedule 4 drugs include hallucinogens such as cannabis, cannabis resin, bufotenine, mescaline, lysergic acid and similar substances.

What is **alcoholism** *and how common is it?*

Alcoholism refers to those dependent on alcohol to such an extent as to produce physical or mental ill-health or interference with interpersonal relationships and normal socio-economic functioning. The World Health Organisation recognises these factors in its definition and includes also those showing the prodromal signs of such development.

The incidence of alcoholism in England and Wales is said to be about one per cent. Accurate statistics are difficult to obtain since hospital admissions include mainly alcoholics with physical or mental complications. Similarly, police figures for charges attributable to drinking apply to a very highly selected group, many of whom are not true alcoholics. Alcoholism is commoner in men.

Discuss **Jellinek's contribution** *to the study of alcoholism*

1. Jellinek produced a *formula* which attempts to estimate the incidence of alcoholism with physical complications. It is based

on several assumptions and utilises such data as percentage contribution of alcoholism to a particular disease, the total number of deaths from that disease, etc. The formula is of limited practical value.

2. *Classification.* Jellinek considers alcoholism to be a generic term which includes a large number of species, i.e. types of alcoholism (in all of which some psychiatric vulnerability is present).

(*a*) alpha. No loss of control over alcohol intake, and no inability to abstain. Mainly psychological dependence.

(*b*) beta. Physical complications, e.g. cirrhosis, but no psychological or physical dependence.

(*c*) gamma. Dependence (psychological and physical) with loss of control and symptoms on withdrawal.

(*d*) delta. Dependent, and inability to abstain, with no loss of control.

(*e*) epsilon. The bout drinker (dipsomaniac).

Discuss the **aetiology** of alcoholism

1. *Physiological.* Various physical abnormalities have been sought to try and explain the alcoholic's predilection for alcohol on the basis of abnormal tissue metabolism. Alcoholics have often been divided into primary or secondary groups. It is then hypothesised that the primary (or addictive) alcoholic has some constitutional physical predisposition leading to a need to imbibe alcohol to excess. Vitamin deficiency, abnormal mineral metabolism and enzymes have been implicated, but with no conclusive results. Vitamin and other deficits in alcoholics are always secondary to the alcoholism itself.

2. *Psychological.* Drinking is often referred to as being secondary or symptomatic. This indicates that the alcoholic drinks to alleviate some discomfort. The latter may be anxiety, depression, etc., and the personality of the alcoholic is frequently, if not always, vulnerable.

Psychoanalytic views include the ability of alcohol to bolster the ego of individuals who tolerate frustration poorly; alcohol dependence is a complication of oral dependence, latent homosexuality and an unconscious drive towards self-destruction; alcohol is a substitute for mothers' milk.

Learning theory has contributed to the understanding of alcoholism at the purely behavioural level. It was shown that animals could be protected from 'experimental neuroses' by alcohol. More recently, learning theory models have been constructed. Alcohol is accordingly regarded as a means of producing pleasant sensations, providing drinking with its own reward. Thus each time the alcoholic drinks, the reward reinforces his drinking habit.

3. *Socio-cultural.* There are wide variations in the incidence of alcoholism among different cultures and races, e.g. it is frequent in the Irish and infrequent in Jews. Availability and price are other factors, which probably explain the high incidence in the wine-producing countries of Europe. Also, society's attitude to the drinker must be an important factor. Alcoholism is an occupational hazard among publicans, salesmen and businessmen. In the vulnerable personality, social drinking can escalate to pathological drinking under the influence of sub-cultural or occupational pressures.

4. *Sex.* Males are far more prone to alcoholism than females, but female alcoholics are more difficult to treat.

5. *Family.* Alcoholics are more likely to derive from large families and they tend to be the younger members. Among male alcoholics, there is a preponderance of those who are either unmarried, widowers or separated from their wives. The last, can be a cause or effect of the drinking.

What are the **clinical features** *of alcohol dependence?*

1. *Physical or mental complications* of alcoholism, e.g. peripheral neuropathy, large liver, withdrawal signs, memory impairment.

2. *Other physical signs* may include conjunctivitis, bronchitis, and gastritis as evidenced by morning vomiting.

3. *Amnesias*—'blackouts'—are often a sinister development in the alcoholic's history.

4. *Change in drinking habits*, e.g. the necessity of drinking first thing in the morning, the development of a craving for alcohol; change of beverage may occur in some alcoholics because of a need to imbibe something more potent (i.e. tolerance to the usual dose of alcohol developing) or owing to financial considerations.

5. *Deterioration in habits.* The patient may spend progressively larger amounts of money on alcohol and this may lead to socio-economic deterioration, or marital separation, these factors being potentiated if he becomes unemployed because of inefficiency, absenteeism or intoxication. He may become careless and repeatedly injure himself. Finally, a loss of personal pride often sets in, and a doss-house or 'Skid Row' existence ensues.

6. *Emotional or personality changes.* Irritability, depression and suspiciousness are common features in the chronic alcoholic and pathological jealousy (directed at the wife) may occur. A noisy, boisterous euphoria is sometimes the mood, but the affect tends ultimately to become shallow, insincere and finally flat.

Organic personality changes are important psychiatric complications of chronic alcoholism and occur insidiously over the years (see below).

Write short notes on the **physical complications of alcoholism**

1. *Wernicke's encephalopathy.* This acute brain disturbance occurs on the basis of a deficiency of vitamin B_1 (thiamine). Malnutrition is the commonest cause, although repeated vomiting may also play a part. The patient becomes confused and unsteady in his gait (ataxia) and gives evidence of midbrain damage, e.g. complains of double vision and demonstrates paralysis of eye movements. If confusion is not noted, memory impairment is usually obvious, and is evident on recovery.

Pathological changes consist of congestion, necrosis and haemorrhage in the region of the mammillary bodies and hypothalamus.

Peripheral neuritis is almost invariably present.

2. *Peripheral neuritis or neuropathy.* This can be sensory, motor or mixed. Thiamine deficiency is thought to be one of the commoner aetiological factors.

3. *Alcoholic myopathy.* This is characterised by gradual weakness and atrophy of the proximal muscles.

4. *Rare brain degenerations.* (*a*) Cerebellar degeneration. (*b*) Marchiafava-Bignami disease. Described in Italian wine-drinkers, but can rarely occur in any form of alcoholism, especially if associated with vitamin deficiency and malnutrition. Patho-

logical changes occur in the corpus callosum. The patient may have epileptic fits. (*c*) Demyelination of brain-stem.

5. *Heart*. (*a*) Alcoholic cardiomyopathy. The myocardium is diseased, and the condition may be confused with coronary heart disease. Does not respond to treatment with thiamine. (*b*) 'Beri-beri' heart. This is less serious than the above, and responds to thiamine.

6. *Liver*. Hepatic *cirrhosis* is a very common complication of chronic alcoholism, although it remains uncertain whether faulty diet or toxic factors are responsible for the fatty infiltration of the liver. Liver damage may itself lead to further complications, e.g. *portal-systemic encephalopathy*. In this condition, physical features, e.g. tremor, focal neurological signs and clouding of consciousness, may present themselves. Psychiatric sequelae may also be prominent, e.g. personality changes, irritability, apathy or depression.

Which psychiatric conditions are associated with **withdrawal of alcohol?**

1. *Delirium tremens*. This acute psychosis follows a period of abstinence from alcohol, e.g. following a drinking binge or post-operatively. There may be prodromal features such as trembling, restlessness and insomnia. The patient exhibits clouding of consciousness and misinterprets his environment . This pro-gresses to hallucinations (visual and occasionally auditory), paranoid ideas and sometimes terror, with persecutory delusions. The patient is hyperactive and may have fits. On examination, there is tremor and often peripheral neuropathy. Infection and vitamin depletion are contributory factors.

2. *Fits*. Often associated with the D.T.s

3. *'Shakes'*, which are often referred to as tremulous state or withdrawal tremor. They occur in the morning and the patient finds that taking a drink relieves this symptom. ('The hair of the dog that bit.')

4. *Alcoholic hallucinations*. Auditory hallucinations occur in the absence of confusion, and in association with paranoid ideas. In the chronic state it may resemble paranoid schizophrenia.

Discuss the **psychiatric complications** *of alcoholism*

In addition to withdrawal syndromes, chronic alcoholics are

prone to exhibit certain mental illnesses which may or may not be associated with physical complications. Some of the features of alcoholic dependence are usually discernible.

Korsakoff's psychosis. This may develop insidiously or follow an attack of delirium tremens or Wernicke's encephalopathy. It is characterised by poor memory for recent events, confabulation, disorientation, suggestibility and emotional disturbances such as lability, flatness or benign euphoria. This syndrome was originally described in an alcoholic with peripheral neuritis and is now frequently referred to as the Korsakoff or Dysmnesic Syndrome, with memory impairment as the primary disability. It can also be caused by head injury, arteriosclerosis, cerebral neoplasm, prolonged anoxia and brain operations.

Pathological changes occur in the mammillary bodies.

Personality changes are frequent among chronic alcoholics. Thinking becomes slow and laboured and talk is circumstantial with free use of clichés. The content usually concerns the past. Judgment becomes impaired and general grasp is poor, on account of difficulty in learning new information. There are usually associated emotional changes, e.g. fatuous bonhomie, labile emotional display or undue irritability. Depression and consequently suicide are frequent in alcoholics, but their occurrence do not depend on the development of personality deterioration. *Dementia* is the end-stage of organic personality changes. In the early stage there is defective memory for recent events and the patient's ability to learn new material diminishes progressively. Affect deteriorates further, culminating in apathy and flattened emotional response, while initiative and ability to lead an independent existence are lost.

A few alcoholics pass through the Korsakoff state before dementing.

Paranoid reactions and psychoses occur frequently in the form of *pathological jealousy*, the male alcoholic often becoming impotent in an already deteriorating marital situation. They may also be part of an *alcoholic hallucinosis*.

What is meant by **dipsomania?**

This term refers to periodic drinking of excessive amounts of alcohol. These bouts may coincide with episodes of depression or other periodic mental abnormalities. During them, the alcoholic completely loses control of his drinking habits. At other times he may be able to abstain completely.

What is meant by **pathological intoxication?**

Some individuals, e.g. after a head injury, or epileptics and psychopaths, may be very susceptible to alcohol. Such patients may become violent and later have no recollection of the event, as in states of epileptic automatism, and it is probably significant that most have abnormal EEGs.

Give an outline of the **treatment** of alcoholism

Alcoholics may require treatment for withdrawal symptoms, dependence on alcohol, for the physical or psychiatric complications, or for the original psychiatric illness such as depression or anxiety state.

Admission to hospital is generally advisable and is essential if *withdrawal* symptoms are present. Delirium tremens is the most severe withdrawal syndrome and should be treated with bed rest and tranquillisers. Haloperidol is usually effective but in the emergency treatment of D.T.s chlordiazepoxide (Librium) and diazepam (Valium) act more quickly when given intravenously. Attention to fluid and electrolytes is as important as any of the other measures and large doses of vitamins given intravenously or intramuscularly in the form of 'parentrovite' are indicated. Therapy with *vitamins* especially of the 'B' group, though frequently advised for many forms of alcoholism, are in no way specific, but should be given where there is reason to believe that the patient is depleted of such vitamins, e.g. in Wernicke's encephalopathy, the 'beri-beri' type of heart complication, and in the multiple dietary deficits to which alcoholics are prone.

The treatment of *alcoholic dependence* is that of the underlying condition, coupled with advice to the patient to abstain completely. Results of any treatment are poor if the patient is not sufficiently well motivated. The following measures are available:

1. *Psychotherapy* is often helpful in elucidating the conflicts and anxiety which are contributing to the patient's alcoholism. A superficial supportive approach can be effective, particularly if it

extends to the patient's family, who in turn may become more supportive to the patient. A helpful spouse is the best prognostic factor.

2. *Group therapy* is used to a large extent, especially in the form of Alcoholics Anonymous. It can also be given on an out-patient basis for a prolonged period, thus maintaining essential contact between patient and hospital.

3. *Alcoholics Anonymous.* This lay organisation has branches and meetings in most parts of the country, and provides advice, support and encouragement on group lines for alcoholics by abstaining alcoholics.

4. *Hostels.* There are a few which cater for the needs of some alcoholics by providing a supportive environment for a prolonged period, with access if necessary to active treatment. These are especially useful for the alcoholic who has deteriorated socially, is derelict, unemployed and with no stable home. Rehabilitation is often necessary for such chronic alcoholics who have become unemployed and alienated from their relatives.

5. *Behaviour therapy*

Aversion therapy. The aim is to set up an anti-alcohol conditioned response in the patient, the unconditioned stimulus being an emetic or an electric shock. Apomorphine or emetine injections can be given as the emetic. *Antabuse* (disulfiram), which is available in tablet form, when taken regularly, leads to abnormal and unpleasant reactions to alcohol. It blocks the oxidation of alcohol at the acetaldehyde level, leading to the accumulation of the latter in the body after alcohol is taken. A few test reactions with alcohol are given while the patient is still in hospital, but it can only be successful if the patient takes his tablets regularly, and a supportive relative at home is almost essential. (Abstem is a drug with a similar action to Antabuse.)

Write a note on the action of **barbiturates and barbiturate addiction**

Barbiturates produce central depression varying from mild sedation to deep anaesthesia, dependent only upon the dose of the drug and the method of administration. Mild sedation is produced by small doses while large doses produce sleep, and the drug is usually prescribed as a hypnotic. The EEG record is characteristically fast. Barbiturates have achieved immense popularity and are distributed widely, consequently they are the commonest means of attempting suicide although second to carbon monoxide for successful suicide.

Barbiturates should not be prescribed for psychiatric symptoms such as anxiety, depression, etc., since such patients together with those of unstable personality are particularly prone to drugs of addiction. In addition, as already stated, they are frequently used in suicide attempts.

Acute intoxication with barbiturates produces drowsiness and if the dose is large enough coma may result, particularly if they have been taken together with alcohol or other sedatives. Physical signs include a fall in temperature, pulse rate and respiration rate. Neurological disturbances include ataxia, inco-ordination, nystagmus and flaccidity of tone.

In *chronic intoxication* a picture similar to that of chronic alcoholism occurs with variations in mood, irritability, impairment of judgment and lack of grasp. Ataxia, inco-ordination and dysarthria are accompanying physical signs.

On *withdrawal* or marked decrease in dosage, minor symptoms such as anxiety, tremor, dizziness, slight drop in blood pressure, nausea or insomnia may result, but the most dangerous withdrawal effects are delirium and convulsions of the grand mal type. Barbiturate addiction is often associated with addiction to other drugs, e.g. alcohol and amphetamine.

In *treatment* of barbiturate addiction the dosage must be reduced very slowly to obviate the possibility of withdrawal fits. It is usual to prescribe an anti-convulsant in addition, e.g. epanutin 100 mg. t.d.s. Major tranquillisers such as chlorpromazine are usually given, or alternatively one of the benzdiazapines. Residual depression might well require treatment on its own account. As in the treatment of any addiction, supportive psychotherapy may be necessary.

Discuss opiate addiction

This includes addiction to morphine, heroin and synthetic equivalent drugs. Some addicts belong to the professions, e.g. medical, nursing, dental, etc., which have easy access, but the majority, in recent times, are of psychopathic or otherwise unstable personality and obtain the drug from non-medical sources. Some may simulate abdominal pains to gain admission to hospital in order to obtain supplies. Addiction to morphine and heroin occurs easily because of their analgesic and euphoriant properties, the development of tolerance, and the psychological and physical dependence that readily develops. Addiction may first be recognised only after the patient has been admitted to hospital and when withdrawal signs appear, which is 12 to 48 hours after initial withdrawal and include features such as depression, restlessness, irritability, diarrhoea, salivation, yawning and abdominal pains. The opiate addict exhibits chronic malaise, tremors, small pupils, sluggishness of the gut, decrease in muscular power and in sexual potency. Skin punctures are often in evidence.

Addiction to morphine or heroin is often accompanied by addiction to a stimulating drug such as cocaine or amphetamine.

In *treatment* the gradual withdrawal of the drug is indicated and methadone is often used in the withdrawal process. A major tranquilliser such as chlorpromazine is usually prescribed to cover some of the anxiety and other withdrawal symptoms and subsequently supportive psychotherapy, sometimes in groups, is given. In the treatment of this and other forms of addiction, modified insulin is sometimes used as an adjunct in treatment, especially when there has been considerable weight loss. Continuous narcosis is now being tried in drug centres, but it is too early to evaluate results.

What is a **narcotic antagonist?**

In recent years, the use of such drugs in the treatment of heroin addiction has been explored. Cyclazocine is the most prominent example of this group. It is a synthetic analgesic related to nalorphine, and antagonises both the central and systemic effects of opiates. It can be employed during the withdrawal phase in addicts as an alternative to employing another narcotic such as methadone. Narcotic antagonists have not yet received a long enough trial for results to be regarded as more than preliminary.

Write a note on **cocaine addiction**

Since cocaine is a stimulant, addicts to morphine and heroin use it as an accessory. It used to be sniffed and would cause ulceration of the nose, but nowadays it tends to be taken by injection. It produces elation, excitement, tirelessness, restlessness and increase of energy. Intoxication often leads to hallucinations and delirious states and the characteristic feeling of formication which consists of a form of tactile hallucination, the patient believing that there are insects crawling on his skin. Withdrawal effects do not tend to be marked.

Write a note on **amphetamine addiction**

Amphetamine is a stimulant drug which used to be prescribed for the treatment of depression. It is often taken by addicts as a supplement to their barbiturates or alcohol to produce a euphoriant effect, and thus many unstable personalities and psychopaths become addicted. Addiction may also result from its prescription for depression or as a slimming tablet. Overdosage and intoxication produces restlessness and delirium which may mimic hypomania or mania.

Addiction may produce a psychosis with paranoid delusions and auditory hallucinations, and the clinical picture may resemble paranoid schizophrenia, especially in a young, unstable person. In addition, behavioural disturbances of an anti-social type and other irresponsible behaviour may result. On withdrawal, severe depression or a paranoid psychosis may ensue.

The Drugs (Prevention of Misuse) Act (1964) applied to amphetamines and similar stimulants, and limited the import and possession of such drugs. The new Misuse of Drugs Act (1971) has more recently been introduced and supersedes the earlier Act. (See question on recent legislation on drugs.)

What are the **hallucinogenic drugs?**

These drugs include mescaline, LSD (lysergic acid diethylamide), psilocybin and cannabis (hashish or marihuana). They all enhance sensory, especially visual, perception and often lead to visual hallucinations and produce a dream-like state which may lead to incoherent thoughts, feelings of unreality and depersonalisation. They were used as an adjunct in psychotherapy because of the claim that they enhanced the recall of earlier experiences with the consequent ventilation of emotion, i.e. abreaction. They are now rarely used in therapy because of their relative inefficiency and addiction potential. Because they can produce hallucinations they are often referred to as *psychotomimetic* drugs, and theories to explain the mechanism of functional psychoses such as schizophrenia have been based on the discovery in schizophrenics of abnormal metabolites which are chemically related to the hallucinogens. The case is still unproven chemically and there are also wide discrepancies between the clinical features of schizophrenia and the hallucinatory experiences induced by these drugs.

Cannabis is imported illegally in large quantities and LSD is synthesised in a clandestine manner in the U.K., so that both drugs are subjected to abuse, especially by some young people who experiment with them in search of new experiences.

Although it is technically correct that neither LSD nor cannabis lead to true dependence, they can provoke psychotic states. LSD is by far the more dangerous, since very small doses may precipitate an LSD psychosis, complete with visual and auditory hallucinations and loss of control of behaviour and emotions.

Suicide and murder have been committed under the influence of this drug. There may be a latent period, of anything up to 3 weeks, between ingesting LSD and the report of psychiatric sequelae. Further, the transient hallucinatory state may subside within a matter of hours or days, but leave in its train a more chronic state, with apathy, lack of drive and concentration as well as 'flash-backs'. For some vulnerable individuals this state may persist for months, with consequent disastrous effects on school, work and family.

SECTION 13

PSYCHOPATHIC PERSONALITY

What is a **psychopathic personality?**

There are numerous definitions as, for instance:

1. *Schneider* (1934). P.P.s are those abnormal personalities who suffer from their abnormality or from whose abnormality society suffers.

2. *White* (1935). Psychopathic as a prefix has come to be a wastebasket into which all sorts of things have been thrown. Society has developed machinery—more or less ponderous and creaking and ineffective to be sure, but nevertheless based upon fairly concrete formulations—for handling the so-called insane at one end and the so-called criminal at the other. The psychopaths fall between. They belong to neither group, and they get into either more or less by accident.

3. *Henderson* (1939). The exact term we use is perhaps not very material so long as we define what éxactly we mean, but personally I prefer to use the term psychopathic state because it does not stress unduly either innate or acquired characteristics, and does not imply total mental unsoundness, defect or delinquency, but yet allows for modifications of all of them . . . it is the name we apply to those individuals who conform to a certain intellectual standard, sometimes high, sometimes approaching the realm of defect but not yet amounting to it, who throughout their lives, or from a comparatively early age, have exhibited disorders of conduct of an anti-social or asocial nature, usually of a recurrent or episodic type, which, in many instances, have proved difficult to influence by methods of social, penal and medical care and treatment, and for whom we have no adequate provision of a preventative or curative nature. The inadequacy, deviation or failure to adjust to ordinary social life is not a mere wilfulness or badness which can be threatened or thrashed out of the individual, but constitutes a true illness for which we have no specific explanation.

4. *Cheney* (1934). P.P.s are characterised largely by emotional immaturity or childishness with marked defects of judgment and without evidence of learning by experience. They are prone to impulsive reactions without consideration of others, and to emotional instability with rapid swings from elation to depression, often apparently for trivial reasons. Special features in individual psychopaths are prominent criminal traits, moral deficiency, vagabondage and sexual perversion. Intelligence shown by standard intelligence tests may be normal or superior, but on the other hand, not infrequently a border-line intelligence may be present.

5. *Levine* (1942). They tend to act out their conflicts in social life, instead of developing symptoms of conflict in themselves.

None, however has surpassed that of J. C. Pritchard, the Gloucestershire physician who described the condition in 1835 as 'the moral and active principles of the mind are strongly perverted or depraved; the power of self-government is lost or greatly impaired and the individual is found to be incapable not of talking or reasoning upon any subject proposed to him, but of conducting himself with decency and propriety in the business of life'.

The Mental Health Act (1959) defines a *'psychopathic disorder'* as a persistent disorder or disability of the mind (whether or not including subnormality of intelligence) which results in abnormally aggressive or seriously irresponsible conduct on the part of the patient and requires or is susceptible to treatment.

A feature which many of these definitions omit is the relative or complete *absence of a sense of shame or guilt* associated with the antisocial conduct.

Discuss the **classification** *of psychopathic personalities (personality disorders)*

There are numerous classifications just as there are definitions: under these the commoner are those of:

1. *Kraepelin* (1909-13). The excitable, the unstable, the impulsive, the liars and swindlers, the anti-social, the quarrelsome.

2. *Partridge* (1930). *Inadequate*—(a) insecure, (b) depressive, (c) weak-willed, (d) asthenic. *Egocentric*—(a) contentious, (b) paranoid, (c) explosive, (d) excitable, (e) aggressive. *Criminal*—(a) liars, (b) swindlers, (c) vagabonds, (d) sexual perverts.

3. *Schneider* (1934). (*a*) hyperthymic, (*b*) depressive, (*c*) self-insecure, (*d*) fanatics, (*e*) attention-seeking, (*f*) temperamentally unstable, (*g*) explosive, (*h*) insensitive or anti-social, (*i*) weak-willed, (*j*) asthenic.

4. *Menninger* (1941). (*a*) the predatory, (*b*) the sycophantic, (*c*) the histrionic, (*d*) the façade, (*e*) the transilient.

5. *Henderson* (1939). (*a*) predominantly aggressive, (*b*) predominantly inadequate, (*c*) predominantly creative.

6. *American Psychiatric Association.* (*a*) pathologic sexuality, (*b*) pathologic emotionality, (*c*) asocial or amoral trends.

What is the **aetiology** of psychopathic personality?

A variety of factors have been involved, the commoner ones are:

1. *Constitutional*

Some evidence has been obtained from studies of epileptics and people with brain damage. Impulsive criminals have been investigated with EEG studies and it has been shown that unpremeditated crimes are associated with a high percentage of abnormal records.

2. *Biochemical and endocrine*

Evidence for this has come from studies of the effect of blood sugar on the EEG and on human behaviour, as well as certain psychological difficulties occurring in dysmenorrhoeic women or in those with premenstrual tension. In the latter instances EEG studies have also been confirmatory.

3. *Prenatal and perinatal factors*

These have been defined, mainly in delinquent children, but the evidence is not strong and it has been considered that if these factors play any part in the causation of delinquency it is a very small and indirect one.

4. *Genetic aspects*

Abnormal sex chromosome complements have been found to be five times greater in mental deficiency institutions than in the normal population. Among aggressive patients of large stature a significantly high proportion show the XYY phenomenon (see Section 5).

5. *Psychological*

Psychopathic behaviour has been described by the psycho-analytical school as 'impulse neuroses'. Such individuals have been described as 'hypersexual and hyperinstinctual' and when their feelings are dammed up they tend to eventually explode, frequently into unreliable and antisocial conduct. The rudimentary super-ego in these patients has been constantly pointed out and is alleged to be responsible for the absence of a feeling of shame or guilt and the absence of remorse following the crimes they commit.

With the present accent on behavioural psychology which considers that all aberrant behaviour is maladaptive and due to faulty conditioning, psychopathy is also included and is attributed to faulty learning.

Discuss the **manipulative personality**

This term has been used to describe in psychological terms the sociopath. The key elements of manipulation are: (a) the perception of a conflict of goals between the manipulator and another; (b) the intention to influence the other by employing a deception of some sort; (c) the feeling of exhilaration at having put something over on the other person; and (d) he is aware of these activities and enjoys them and actively seeks or contrives at such situations.

He has an intensive narcissism and can only feel lovable if he is great. He therefore proves himself on other people and shows a contempt for others. Telling the truth has a low priority and he will try and cover himself with deceptions and rationalisations to maintain a good image.

What is **the firesetter syndrome?**

This is a highly determined behavioural complex with important defensive and adaptive aspects. The act is not usually the product of an impulse, but highly determined as it involves ego operations like planning, timing, fantasy elaboration, undoing and identification.

What **treatment** *is available for psychopathic personalities?*

Many methods have been tried from markedly permissive régimes in special institutions based on a therapeutic community to the usual corrective influences supplied by institutional systems such as special institutions and prisons for persistent psychopathic offenders. Some exploit the indeterminate sentence which acts as a deterrent, but this is supplemented with intensive after-care and follow-up, and in countries where the social services are able to cope with this heavy demand the results have been encouraging.

The commonest single factor in recovery from psychopathic behaviour is *maturation* and any manoeuvre which can accelerate maturation is likely to be helpful. Society's various experiments have shown that efforts to promote maturation have not necessarily been more successful with highly trained analytical personnel, and that an experienced prison officer or Borstal Master may have achieved equal, if not greater, success.

Scott has elaborated groups of psychopathic personalities which he feels indicate the type of treatment which is most likely to help. These are:

1. *Trained, but to anti-social standards*

Treatment, restraint, including punishment with advice and assistance.

2. *Reparative behaviour*

Treatment here should be restraint, but psychotherapy may also be needed to cope with the patient's defences.

3. *The untrained offender*

This person is without standards and weak in character, with difficulties stemming from early life. Treatment, therefore, consists of long-term, patient supervision with a background of sanctions. Heavy punishment would be contraindicated.

4. *Rigid fixations*

These are rather stereotyped conditions which do not respond to punishment or treatment and still present a problem to be solved.

SECTION 14

SEX AND ITS DISORDERS

What is meant by **sexual perversion?**

Sexual perversion is a form of sexual behaviour or preoccupation which is other than genital to genital in its final purpose and which the individual prefers to this form of expression. Though such a definition would include masturbation in adolescence or in other circumstances where normal heterosexual experience is unobtainable, it would not be regarded as a perversion provided phantasies are frankly heterosexual.

Discuss **sexual appetite and its disorders**

Normal sexual appetite is almost impossible to define, for, like appetite for food, there are wide variations. Appetites may be *increased* because of:

1. Latent homosexuality in male and female.
2. Febrile states as in early tuberculosis.
3. Manic states in both sexes.
4. Schizophrenic states which may predispose to nymphomanic behaviour.
5. Paranoid states where the latent homosexuality drives male or female to constantly try and prove their sexuality.
6. Drugs.

Diminished appetite may be due to the following factors:

1. Age.
2. Other interests.
3. Latent homosexuality.
4. Loss of interest in partner.
5. Depression.
6. Debilitating diseases.

What are the **commoner clinical varieties** *of sexual perversion?*

1. *Sadism.* The term is derived from the Marquis de Sade (1740-1814), a French writer of obscene novels whose main theses were lust and cruelty.

2. *Masochism.* The term is derived from the name of Leopold von Sacher-Masoch (1836-95), who described men being dominated by women and who in his private life expressed desires that his wife should be unfaithful to him. Sadism and masochism are frequently complex and are present in the same individual. *Flagellation* is the commonest masochistic practice, either self-inflicted or at the hands of others; it also looms large in the fantasies of masochists.

3. *Fetishism.* This is almost exclusively a male perversion and it applies to sexual stimulation by part of the female such as the hair or foot, or an article of clothing. The further removed the stimulating object from the partner's body, the more pronounced the fetishism is said to be, favourite objects being underclothes, stockings, shoes, brassières, and at the beginning of the century, garters. Fetishism has also been attributed to temporal lobe disturbances and it may occur in cerebral tumours in this region.

4. *Transvestism and transsexualism.* A transvestite is a person who prefers to wear clothing belonging to the opposite sex and has a desire to assume the role of that sex. Some claim that all transvestites are homosexuals though this view has not been generally accepted; nevertheless most transvestites desire a sex change in order to make themselves more attractive to partners of their own sex. Transsexuals are those who would prefer to undergo a physical sex change and, in fact, many of them seek surgical treatment or hormone therapy in order to effect this change.

5. *Exhibitionism.* This is the displaying of genitalia, usually for the purpose of sexual gratification, and again is exclusively a male perversion, and should not be confused with strip-tease shows where men are entertained by women; in this instance it is purely a form of entertainment. Three categories are involved:

(*a*) The dullard who is handicapped in his courtship and who uses exhibitionism to promote it.

H

(b) The elderly male with arteriosclerosis or other brain change who lacks control and may be goaded into exposing himself by curious little girls in the park.

(c) Those of good intellect but who have this compulsion, usually to affront or shock the opposite sex, and these are the ones who become the chronic recidivists.

6. *Voyeurism*. This is predominantly a male perversion and is a means of obtaining sexual gratification by looking at sexual organs or others engaged in sexual activity.

7. *Obscenity*. This is the use of words or phrases either by mouth or by writing as a means of achieving sexual excitement or inducing it in others, included in this is the writing on lavatory walls called *graffiti*.

8. *Pornography*. This is really an aspect of voyeurism in that words instead of pictures or scenes are used to provide sexual gratification. It ranges from obscene words designed to shame the listener or reader to literary classics, from graffiti and bawdy songs to the most delicately composed sonnets. As with voyeurism, women are less stimulated by this literature than men.

9. *Coprophilia*. This is extended to urethral erotic perversions as well as anal-erotic ones and in fact the former is the more commonly practised and may account for those men who secrete themselves in female lavatories. They may come to the casualty departments of general hospitals with foreign bodies in the urethra and rectum.

10. *Coprolalia*. This is a combination of coprophilia, exhibitionism and sadism and consists of a compulsion to utter obscenities. Occasionally the impulse is partially controlled and a form of stuttering results, with explosive noises which resemble the obscene words but are prevented from full expression. This condition, when associated with compulsive movements is referred to as the Gilles de la Tourette syndrome. It may also take the form of obscene telephone calls where the listener chosen is invariably female and the caller is male.

11. *Fellatio*. This is oral contact with the male genitalia; *cunnilingus* is oral contact with the female genitalia.

12. *Anolingus*. This is oral contact, usually with the tongue and rectum. It is commonly described in pornographic literature.

13. *Frotteurism*. This is contact with another person in order to obtain sexual satisfaction, usually by rubbing oneself up against them in crowds, crowded stores or in queues.

14. *Bondage*. This is a form of masochism in which erotic pleasure is associated with being humiliated, endangered and enslaved, and with being bound, restrained and rendered helpless to a degree that life is threatened. There is an erotisation of the situation with a general sexual orientation towards homosexuality.

Write a note on **ejaculatio praecox**

Three main types are described:

1. *Habitual*, with strong erections present constantly since adolescence.
2. *Acute onset*, generally with erectional insufficiency occurring in young men, usually in response to specific psychological or psychophysical stress.
3. *Insidious onset*, generally with erectional insufficiency and other evidence of declining sexual responsiveness occurring generally in older men.

Treatment

1. Muscular relaxation for cases with high levels of coital anxiety (Types 1 and 2).
2. Repeated stimulation and interruption according to the technique of Seman. The female partner provides extravaginal stimulation to the instructions of the male when he is fully roused sexually but non-anxious. It is interrupted when the male indicates that orgasm is imminent and when feeling has faded stimulation is again started and the process repeated several times.
   Masters and Johnson recommend a different technique. The female lies on top of the male and when he is about to ejaculate, she firmly pinches the shaft of the penis between her fingers, causing a reflex interruption of orgasm. When it has been averted, intercourse can recommence with further similar interruptions if necessary.

3. Sexual education is helpful in Type 2.
4. Novel and excitatory sexual stimulation is helpful in Type 3.
5. Explanatory talks are generally helpful.

What is meant by **the new impotence?**

Rapid changes in social mores may be reflected in changes in psychiatric symptomatology. Increased sexual freedom of women can induce impotence in the male partner. This is a reversal of former roles: that of the put-upon Victorian woman is now the put-upon man of the 1970s. It does not necessarily reflect the woman's increased need for sexual pleasure but a form of feminine revenge which reinforces the man's castration anxiety.

Write short notes on **impotence** and **frigidity**

Impotence is the partial or total inability of the male to achieve and maintain an erection during sexual intercourse. In overt or latent homosexuals the disability may be total though not necessarily. For example, the Don Juan type may try to deny his latent homosexuality by repeated conquests and may even display hypersexuality.

Some may be impotent in the marital setting but competent with a prostitute or by nourishing prostitution fantasies by getting their partner to dress the part or behave in an uninhibited sexual manner and thus debase herself. Others may require a sado-masochistic relationship to stimulate them.

The commonest form of impotence is the person who is either in a depressive or anxiety state and these generally respond to treatment. Unfortunately many middle-aged men seek extra-marital affairs to revitalise a flagging libido and thus complicate the picture and impede recovery.

Frigidity. This too can be based on a latent homosexuality but is most commonly associated with anxiety. Many patients with phobic anxiety are frigid and are rendered symptom-free when the phobic state is successfully treated. Where the frigidity is not associated with anxiety or depression, it frequently responds to local measures such as recommended for the treatment for dyspareunia (see Section 8).

Discuss **homosexuality**

Homosexuality is a sexual orientation to a member of the same sex and it need not necessarily imply physical contact; in fact most homosexuals who are aware of their homosexuality do not necessarily indulge in homosexual practices but have a continent relationship with their partner.

Psychopathology. From the psychoanalytical standpoint, castration anxiety is the basis of most cases of male homosexuality. There is an awareness that the female has no penis and this in itself implies a threat of castration which may be transferred to the female genitalia. The choice of a male partner by the male may be due to over-identification with the mother, which may encourage the patient to seek out adolescents so that he can adopt the maternal role towards someone he can regard as himself. Alternatively it may take the form of trying to obtain sexual satisfaction in the manner of the mother. This attitude could also be interpreted as a passive-receptive one to the father and through anal intercourse it can also represent an attempt at symbolic castration of the father with reduction in the patient's own castration anxiety.

Biological factors. It has been shown by Tinbergen that the black-headed gull's 'escape' and 'attack' behaviour during early territorial squabbles is frequently carried over into mating with sexual responses instead of combative ones becoming manifest. Males would mount males at times of sexual frustration such as the end of the season, particularly when the crouching position of one bird had triggered off this behaviour, although the assaulted male would repel the advance. In monkey colonies, males may 'present' to the dominant monkey, who may accept this offer of anal intercourse. There is a very large step from this type of animal behaviour to homosexuality in human beings. Other biological aspects such as chromosome studies and somatotyping have not revealed any difference between homosexuals and heterosexuals.

Genetic aspects. Although at one time it was considered that there was strong genetic evidence for homosexuality, this has now been discounted.

Social factors. Homosexual behaviour can be influenced by environment, and men in captivity, either in prisons, prisoner-of-war camps or on lonely stations in war service, developed very strong homosexual attachments. A climate which favours or promotes homosexual behaviour may also stimulate a person who was hitherto heterosexual in his orientation to indulge in homosexual activities. Kinsey has rated homosexuals on a seven-point scale and the place in the scale depends upon the amount of overt homosexual commitment and the psychic reaction to sex factors. It is impossible to divide people into two categories, homosexual and heterosexual, as people may move from one to the other, and many are bisexual.

From the psychoanalytical standpoint there are three types of homosexual. (1) *The repressed homosexual*; he or she is the person who has emerged from early homosexual orientation in childhood to full heterosexuality. (2) *The latent homosexual*: he or she is the person who has not completely emerged to full heterosexuality but whose homosexuality is not given full expression and is only in latent form, and this can be sublimated into various activities. There is usually a reflection of homosexual orientation in that they prefer the company of their own sex or lead a celibate existence. (3) *The overt homosexual*: this occurs when the individual is unable to achieve any heterosexual relationship and his sexual object is someone of the same sex, but this does not necessarily mean that he or she indulges in homosexual practices. Female and male are equally vulnerable.

What **treatment** is available for homosexuality and other perversions?

There are three major categories. (1) Psychotherapy of an analytical nature which in well-motivated patients can be successful and until recently was the treatment of choice, and (2) Behaviour therapy, which is usually a form of de-conditioning, particularly of an aversion nature. (3) Drugs: these are most commonly used for the treatment of the male homosexual where stilboestrol is given and also ethinyl oestradiol. Side-effects can be unpleasant and may aggravate the condition in that they can produce enlargement of the breasts and may promote some to become transsexual in their orientation.

Discuss the use of **cyproterone acetate in deviant hypersexuality**

This is a powerful synthetic anti-androgen and progestogen

with antigonadotrophic effects. Dosage is 100 mg. daily in a single morning dose. After 7 days' medication a person with uncontrollable deviant sexual behaviour (attempted incest, homosexuality, transvestism, fetishism and compulsive masturbation) was unable to masturbate to orgasm and ejaculation. There have been no undesirable side-effects or toxic features reported and no evidence of feminisation, and both clinical and endocrine effects were completely reversible in three weeks.

What is the place of **electric aversion therapy** *in the treatment of pathological sexuality?*

· Shocks are given to the forearm from a battery-operated shock box, the level of the shock being decided by the patient. Erections are measured by a penis plethysmograph and subjects are given two sessions daily for 20–30 sessions. With highly motivated patients, 15 per cent were free of their perversion after one year and 57 per cent claimed they had improved. Transvestites, fetishists and sadomasochists improved most, but transsexuals and homosexuals did badly.

Discuss the **legal aspects of homosexuality**

It is a matter which frequently excites considerable controversy in a society in that many people are permissive; others are very repressive and restrictive. Until very recently all homosexual behaviour was illegal and punishable, but under the Homosexual Act (1967) homosexual behaviour between two consenting adults, after the age of 21, in private, is now permitted. Apart from the reductions in prosecutions because of the permissiveness of the Act, there is no evidence that it has contributed to the alleviation or treatment of the problem. It may well have encouraged it, for homosexuality can be contagious and with propaganda it can penetrate into areas of society which were previously non-receptive. It may also deter some from seeking treatment as they no longer have to face legal disapproval. It has also had an impact on public entertainment where flamboyant homosexual attitudes are now portrayed. Revulsion is setting in and 'queer bashing' has become a diversionary exercise for wayward youths and lives have already been lost. It would appear that if government passes more permissive legislation than society is prepared to accept, it can breed reactions more sinister than the previous legislation which contained the problem and did not affront society unduly.

SECTION 15

SOCIAL PSYCHIATRY

What is meant by **social psychiatry?**

This includes all those facets of psychiatry which have social implications such as community care and public health measures including legislation and hospital development. The concept is of relatively recent origin and depends on an appreciation of environmental factors which may influence the onset and prolongation of mental disorders. Until the Second World War the treatment and care of the mentally ill was largely confined to institutions and social manipulation was not a prominent feature. With the incorporation of the principles of Adlerian psychology into general psychiatry a new impulse was given to social manipulation and there is now considerable activity in terms of field studies and experiments in the social aspects of mental illness.

Describe **recent developments** *in social psychiatry*

These can be divided into two: (1) inside the mental hospital and (2) outside the mental hospital.

Inside the mental hospital a variety of measures have been instituted such as:

(*a*) *The breaking up of the mental hospital*: this arose largely out of the unwieldy size of these structures, e.g. in some countries institutions have risen to a patient population of 10,000. Breakdown in size was still in the same framework and led to a larger number of smaller units, with a more intimate appreciation of the patient's problems.

(*b*) *Administrative therapy*: this defines the role of the medical superintendent in the modern mental hospital, and has been defined as the art of treating psychiatric patients in a mental hospital by administrative action. As group therapy has developed from individual therapy so, some claim, administrative therapy is treatment of a much larger group—the hospital.

(*c*) The *therapeutic community*: this derives from the experiment

222

of Maxwell Jones in his efforts to rehabilitate the hitherto incorrigible psychopath by trying to develop a group morality which would prove acceptable. It depends upon a permissive atmosphere pervading the hospital with the authority structure 'flattened' in such a way as to allow patients and staff members with lesser responsibilities to share authority. There is a blurring of staff roles and freer channels of communication. Much of the time is given to making the patient increasingly aware of the effect of his behaviour on other people and therefore he obtains some degree of social insight. It has achieved considerable popularity, but attempts to validate its efficiency as against other forms of psychiatric treatment have not shown it to be of any advantage. There is no uniformity in its practice and one therapeutic community differs from another depending on the type of patient and differences in staff.

(d) *Industrial therapy*: this is the name given to a variety of measures designed to fit the long-stay patient in the mental hospital for work in the community, therefore it largely replaces the occupational therapy department and many mental hospitals now have quite large industrial concerns staffed entirely by patients. It was born out of expediency in that many psychiatric patients were not suitable for industrial rehabilitation units and something specially tailored for their needs was required. The enthusiasm of the organisers has helped to wipe off a backlog of patients who otherwise may not have been rehabilitated, but the hard core problems may prove much more difficult to shift. In addition these measures often depend on an expanding economy with full employment, and the fluctuations of the market may at times prove a very serious obstacle.

(e) *Expansion of services*: some mental hospitals have acquired a 'new look'. This has been largely due to capital expenditure in the establishment of an EEG department which serves the local general hospital as well as the psychiatric hospital, the provision of a child psychiatric unit with paediatric associations, and laboratories which could act as a central laboratory service. Other additions have been geriatric, epileptic and neurosurgical units. The most logical form of expansion is a balanced hospital community where each unit has its part to play and they are all interdependent.

(*f*) The *open door*: this is a recurring theme in mental hospital administration. Patients over the years have been alternately released or locked up, and the present trend is to unlock the doors. Some claim that they run entirely open-door hospitals, in that patients are free to come and go as they please. There are disadvantages in that it can mean too early discharge of patients who should not be allowed to leave the hospital and the inadequate supervision of some infirm senile patients who, because of the open door and lack of nursing supervision, may wander out to their danger. There can be no substitute for the accurate clinical assessment of the needs of each patient.

(*g*) The *team system*: this is an extension of the breaking up of the mental hospital, but in addition departs from previous arrangements when a particular doctor confined his work to the male or female section of the hospital. This allows the psychiatrist to supervise treatment from initial referral, through the treatment unit, to the follow-up clinic, ensuring continuity of care; it also helps to reduce the overall authority of the medical superintendent by giving each team in the hospital its own autonomy.

Developments outside the mental hospital

(*a*) Studies of discharged patients from mental hospital: information derived from these studies helps to assess the impact of long hospital stay on patients and their social liability when discharged. It also gives some indication of community tolerance of those patients who may have been discharged prematurely, or should not have been discharged at all. Information is also coming through as to the best milieu for these discharged patients in that those schizophrenic patients who stay with siblings or in lodgings seem to do better than those who went to parents, wives or large hostels. They also help to highlight the importance of support in the community once the patient has been discharged from hospital.

(*b*) Hostel accommodation: the development of hostels for discharged patients has permitted a much larger number to leave the mental hospital and lead a relatively normal life in the community. These have been described as psychiatric half-way hostels and in those communities where these have been provided there has been less need for the large number of hospital beds, and economically and socially it has proved a very desirable measure. In areas where there is a dearth of hostels, or none at all, the old institutional situation tends to be perpetuated.

(c) Day-hospitals: these have been in operation in Britain for more than 20 years and are assuming a permanent role in the rehabilitation and treatment of mental illness. As most mentally ill patients are ambulatory and can attend hospital for their treatment it makes it possible to treat larger numbers of patients without having to build extra in-patient accommodation. Approximately three day-hospital patients can be treated for the cost of one in-patient, and so on economic grounds this is a decided advantage. In addition it can be much more flexibly used than in-patient accommodation in that the patients may attend for only one, two or three days a week and can be gradually weaned from the support of the day-hospital.

Most physical and psychological treatment used in psychiatry can be given at the day-hospital and the patient is not divorced from his family or the community, so there are social as well as economic advantages. The type of patient selected is equally important and the day-hospital should not be seen as the means of unloading a chronic population because this would destroy its therapeutic value for those with readily recoverable conditions. The day-hospital should, therefore, be seen as the extension of an active in-patient department and not as a special independent unit. Treatment at the day-hospital should be by the same psychiatrist under whom they may have been admitted.

(d) Out-patient departments: these can range from a session held once a week at the mental hospital or in a nearby general hospital, to a fully equipped unit with all facilities for treatment, including occupational therapy department, psychological laboratory, group therapy and out-patient social club. If the out-patient unit is given full support, a psychiatric service can become a small in-patient unit attached to a very busy out-patient and day-hospital service.

(e) The district mental health service: this is firmly based on the mental hospital which, with liaison with neighbouring local authorities, can range over the whole area of hospital and other psychiatric services. It depends on domiciliary visiting by the psychiatrists and an adequate quota of social workers to supervise the discharged patients and, if possible, prevent admission. Such services can help to keep down the number of elderly people admitted to hospital by tackling family rejection as soon as it arises.

(*f*) Community care: this is very close in its conception to the District Mental Health Service, but is more closely linked to the Local Authority through the Medical Officer of Health. It has been given an extra impetus by the Mental Health Act (1959) which considers the local authority responsible for the prophylaxis and after-care of mental illness and although this duty is not yet mandatory it may well become so.

Positive indications for community care rest on a firm diagnosis of mild to moderate illness which can be adequately treated outside hospital with local facilities. It consists of modifying domestic, financial and other environmental stress without having to remove the patient. Community tolerance of the mentally ill is a vital factor in the success of these services, for there is a danger that this tolerance may be stretched to breaking point and produce rejection by the community.

(*g*) The mental welfare officer: psychiatrists have brought the Mental Welfare Officer into the psychiatric clinic. They have used him almost as they would use a psychiatric social worker; with the minimum of formality he can do quite a lot of the work that normally falls to the psychiatric social worker. He can assess the chances of getting the patient a house or a job. He knows the district well in which the patient lives, its cultures and its social mores, and he usually knows whether there is mental illness or deficiency in the family, who is in debt, or behind with the rent, or which relative is in jail. It is this prophylactic aspect of the Mental Welfare Officer which is particularly useful. Recent re-organisation of Welfare Services has replaced the Mental Welfare Officer by a 'generic' social worker with consequent deterioration in the service.

What is the role of the psychiatric unit in the general hospital?

This is a relatively new development in psychiatry and has followed largely on modern methods of treatment which by their success have made most forms of mental illness readily recoverable and a stay in hospital reasonably short. This has approximated psychiatry as a specialty in a general hospital to many other specialties. Relatively few beds are required and these beds are intensively worked and can therefore do much more than a very large unit where the tempo is slower and the ancillary services less well developed. The advantages are not all on the side of the psychiatric unit for the general hospital has also benefited in the following ways:

1. It has brought within its walls a branch of medicine which has to cater for the needs of patients who are not bed-ridden and the other branches of medicine are realising that many of their patients are in the same category and that the psychiatrists can help them in planning their day.

2. It ensures a full-time psychiatric service for the general hospital, with trained personnel immediately available and not based on a mental hospital which may be many miles away.

3. This service extends to the out-patient department, where large numbers of patients referred for medical and surgical opinion are really suffering from mental disturbance.

4. Physical illness does not confer immunity to mental illness, and vice versa, and many patients who may have to be admitted as a psychiatric emergency, are really suffering from the effects of physical illness.

5. The psychiatric department, by introducing the psychological laboratory, a well-supervised occupational therapy department and the concept of the day hospital, brings services to the general hospital which are needed by other specialties.

6. A doctor, whatever his work, is under constant training and a psychiatric department in a general hospital permits a two-way exchange of experiences and instruction which is to the advantage of all.

7. Nursing staff are now expected to get experience of the psychiatric patient, and while a number of general hospitals second student nurses to mental hospitals, a much better arrangement is to have one comprehensive school which caters for all aspects of a nurse's training. A general hospital unit is then put on the same basis as any other branch of nursing and does not divorce the nurse from her contemporaries and tutors. It is also a more suitable place to train the nurse for the future units in psychiatry which are going to be mainly housed in general hospitals.

8. The patients and their relatives should not be expected to go to a different place when treatment can very easily be made available where all other patients are treated. To accentuate this individual difference is artificial and unkind.

Discuss the psychiatric aspects of **geriatrics**

The increase in the aged population and the difficulty in finding accommodation for them in institutions has tended to produce a pessimistic view among workers in the field which the situation may not entirely warrant. Ninety-five per cent of the aged are still living outside institutions and the bonds within most families are strong and enduring. There is however a large marginal group, whose adjustment if undermined would swamp the welfare services. A major factor therefore in the psycho-geriatric problem is family rejection and whatever effort may be made for the treatment of the patient the most important efforts must be directed towards preventing this in the family situation. Once rejection is fully established, almost nothing will alter it.

What measures could be instituted **to prevent rejection?**

Temporary admission to hospital may permit the relatives to have a holiday and thus provide the necessary relief to ensure that the patient may continue to live for the rest of the year in his own home. Day-hospitals are also useful in that they relieve the family of the day-time supervision of the patient and permit the woman of the house to go out to work. Day-centres can cater for the special needs of the aged and many of these are now staffed by both voluntary workers and the local authority. Instead, therefore, of providing more and more residential accommodation for old people, it would be more logical to provide more community services, day-centres, and short-stay in-patient units, so as to give expert help with potential psychiatric illness as early as possible. Hospital and welfare workers, by the very nature of their work, are unaware of the variety of measures which society itself has designed with a 95 per cent success rate. These may be just as worthy of study as the failures.

What is the relationship between **social class and mental illness?**

Social class is usually divided into the five groups as drawn up by the Registrar General. These are (1) professional, business and administration, (2) management and some professional, (3) skilled occupations (manual and clerical), (4) partly-skilled occupations, and (5) unskilled occupations. Studies have shown that schizophrenic patients tend to sediment in groups 4 and 5 and this has been attributed by some to a 'drift' theory in that these patients have deteriorated socially and reach a lower social class because of their mental state. Most studies of the incidence of mental illness are based on those patients who are admitted to mental hospitals. Yet higher social classes and income groups may 'underpin' their unfortunate relatives either by remittance or by some arrangement whereby they are comfortably lodged and cared for. To get a more realistic appreciation of the true social incidence of schizophrenia every private hotel and boarding house should be scrutinised, but by then, the resources of social class 1 and 2 will have found other solutions which may be even more out of range of the sociologists.

Manic and depressive psychoses, and anxiety and severe obsessional states tend to cluster in social class 3 and above. This could be explained by the strong super-ego aspects in these conditions which ensure a conscientiousness and devotion to duty which place these people, when well, in a category which makes them highly desirable in the labour market, and thus ensure them a higher social class.

What is meant by family care or foster-family care?

This is a system which has a very ancient history and in Europe had its origin in Gheel, Belgium. This was the site of a shrine to an Irish princess, and in ancient days pilgrims, many of them insane, visited the shrine and stayed and were looked after by families near by. A colony was eventually established and then a small hospital, and now large numbers of psychiatric patients are treated there and looked after by the villagers. There are many other less well-known examples of this form of care and it is particularly effective in cases of mental subnormality.

Discuss the admission of the children to the psychiatric hospitals where their mothers are patients

This is now a familiar sight and was probably initiated in cases of puerperal psychoses, and in cases where it was either impossible for the new-born child to be looked after apart from its mother, or when it was felt that the mother would benefit from the presence of the child. Initially it would appear that there are many advantages in having the child in with the mother though there has been no evidence to date that there is any difference in the progress of the mother or in the development of the child where the baby was not admitted to hospital. Whenever it is possible, it would appear to be a reasonable thing to do if only on humanitarian grounds, although there are some instances, though rare, where it would be entirely inappropriate for the child to be admitted with the mother because of her mental state.

Discuss mental illness in a new town

There have been several studies recently of these problems, examining incidence, the nature of breakdown and comparisons with similar groups in the older areas from whence the patients were transferred. Various statements have been made about the psychiatric hazards of living in tall blocks of flats as opposed to living nearer the ground, and of the social isolation of housing estates and the like. Evaluation of the data such as has been collected is extremely difficult and the field is still a very open one.

How does social mobility affect psychiatric illness?

Lower social groups tend to have a higher percentage of organic psychoses, psychosomatic problems, functional psychoses, character disorders, alcoholism, dissocial behaviour, hypochondriasis, dependency and schizophrenia. Much of the data is derived from mental hospital admissions but these can be misleading for their clientele is largely drawn from the lower social groups and do not give us much information about the incidence of these problems in the rest of society. It does not therefore mean that if a person moves downwards socially that he is more likely to develop any of these problems; it could be argued that he moved downwards because he had already developed the problem.

Nevertheless, social mobility, particularly upwards, does imply stresses such as extra responsibility, making new social contacts, breaking with old, new hobbies, change of house, and many other changes which some may find too burdensome. It could expose a hitherto abstemious housewife to the cocktail party and alcoholism; to a different mores where sexual adventure is encouraged

and for which she is emotionally unsuited; to the shallow relationships of middle-class suburbia, while she longs for the strong
emotional ties of her working-class background. It may strain
the marital bonds in that the husband is living a different life with
expense account restaurants, hotels and travel which she has been
brought up to view with suspicion if not with hostility. Children
identify more readily with the new environment and this may add
to the mother's estrangement and she may lack the ability to
verbalise her problem and seek the help she needs.

Discuss **mental health and social policy**

In a welfare state when large sums of public money are being
used to provide mental health services it is natural that the
authorities should plan mental health services. Such plans need
not necessarily be advantageous and mistakes have been, and no
doubt will continue to be made and each measure should be
carefully evaluated. Legislation such as the Mental Health Act,
although hailed as enlightened, has shown after a year or two of
operation to have gross defects and, indeed, disadvantages over the
older Acts which it had replaced. Similarly, arrangements for
hospital admissions and the delineation of catchment areas may be
quite reactionary in their concepts. Vested interests such as those
associated with large institutions may overrule more enlightened
experiments which do not have their backing. Because of this
there is a tendency to perpetuate old failures, and new ideas,
though modest, do not inspire the senior planners and are often
not given the encouragement they deserve while large, costly and
sometimes completely inappropriate schemes are given official
backing. Psychiatric illness and an egalitarian approach where
similar facilities are provided for all, may be entirely inappropriate
because there is a strong tendency in this type of illness for people
to seek help from individuals rather than from institutions.

Social changes may influence the incidence of mental disorder
and this has been apparent in dementia paralytica and alcoholism
and provision for the treatment of these patients on a national
scale does mean national planning. On the other hand, in many
forms of psychiatric illness, there is gross discrepancy between
disability and symptomatology and where symptomatology is
present without disability it is not necessarily the illness one is

dealing with but a form of communication, and it is still to be decided whether psychiatric treatment is the best way of dealing with the problems which have inspired this form of communication.

There is a tendency to regard families with problems as problem families and recently the Seebohm Report has advocated the co-ordination of all social services on the assumption that the 'community' whether it be a mining village, an industrial town, a market town, a dormitory suburb or a cathedral city has identical problems which can best be tackled by those who, to date, have ineffectively been involved with problem families. The social worker who has not yet defined her area of competence is to be given responsibility for large sectors where medical and nursing personnel have established high levels of competence. The Mental Welfare Officer and the Day Centre will now come under the Director of Social Service. Unfortunately, social policy has become the plaything of social scientists whose practical experience as far as the needs of society as a whole is concerned is very restricted.

Discuss **cultural factors** in mental health

Differences in incidence of mental illness have been attributed to a variety of factors, but it is becoming increasingly clear that cultural factors play a very important part. This has been shown in the incidence of mental disorders in servicemen where other ranks show an entirely different incidence in certain types of mental illness to that of officers or non-commissioned officers. Similarly, in other cultural groups such as Africans v. Europeans, the incidence say of depressive and anxiety states tends to be much less: even in African groups themselves there are differences between those living in the cities and those living in more primitive surroundings. Cultural factors can produce rather unusual forms of mental illness such as (a) amok and going berserk, (b) latah, which approximates to compulsive movements with echolalia and coprolalia found in Gilles de la Tourette's disease among Europeans, (c) koro (shook yong) which has similarities to a castration fear, and (d) voodoo, which is applied to a form of death when a primitive person has broken a taboo or feels he has been bewitched.

In immigrant communities such as those from the West Indies it has been shown that their previous culture has a 'pathoplastic' effect on their illness, which tends to be coloured by their previous background and superstitions.

What psychiatric problems are found in patients of **no fixed abode?**

In a large urban area there are many who, unable to find work in their own towns, try to find work in the big city. A number are unsuccessful, tend to drift, may be unable to maintain themselves, and, having no lodgings, are classified as of 'no fixed abode'. Those who are admitted to mental hospitals are usually male; unemployed; no family ties; lived at no fixed abode for over a year; more than 50 per cent have a criminal record; are usually compulsory admissions; 76 per cent had previous hospital admissions; one in four discharge themselves against advice; a few are schizophrenics, but the majority are personality disorders some of whom attempt suicide to gain a lodging in hospital. As Jordan (Men Without Homes, 1963) says, 'They have forced themselves upon the attention of society by scavenging, begging, theft, drunkenness and persistent reliance upon public and private charity. They have been regarded as the very epitome of the undeserving poor. . . . The way of life and even the physical setting is remarkably persistent and widespread and the doss-house and missions, the begging, the drinking of cheap fortified wines and non-beverage alcohol and the endless pitiful procession through the police courts. . .'.

The only community they belong to is one which makes no social demands on them and in which debt, crime, neglect, sexual promiscuity, infection and ill-health produce no criticism.

What are the criteria of **problem families?**

These may be listed in the following headings:

1. In a parent: (*a*) low intelligence or mental deficiency, (*b*) mental illness, (*c*) physical handicap or illness which prevents work or permits of light work only—e.g. tuberculosis, heart disease, (*d*) long-continued or recurrent unemployment of main wage-earner from other causes than physical handicap or illness,

(e) excessive drinking, (f) excessive gambling, (g) sexual promiscuity, (h) serving, or has served, a prison sentence, (i) suspected cruelty to or neglect of children, and (j) known cruelty to or neglect of children.

2. Other parental shortcomings: (a) persistent quarrelling, (b) failure to call doctor for major illness, and (c) leaving young children unattended.

3. In a child: (a) repeated hospitalisation of one or more children for gastro-enteritis or respiratory disease, or two or more children for minor accidents, (b) persistent truancy, (c) juvenile delinquency (court cases only), (d) attendance at a child guidance clinic, and (e) under Probation Officer or committed to care by court.

4. Housing: (a) statutory overcrowding, and (b) living in intolerable conditions (while not overcrowded) because of either lack of amenities such as piped water, damp or insanitary conditions, and/or enmity of other occupants of dwelling.

5. Poverty and mismanagement: (a) chronic family debt, (b) lack of minimal necessities of furniture and bedding, (c) inadequate and irregular meals, (d) domestic filth and disorder, (e) wilful damage to property, and (f) lack of, or inadequately maintained, clothing of children.

6. General: (a) unnecessary crowding at night, (b) gross personal uncleanliness, (c) failure to take advantage of necessary help and services proffered, and (d) child or children taken into care other than as the result of court action, and who are frequently taken into or out of care.

What is **mental health consultation?**

Caplan is the main protagonist of the concept of preventive psychiatry for which purpose he has elaborated the *mental health consultation*, even though he admits that there is no evidence to suggest that it is of specific value.

The following characteristics of the process have been defined:

1. Mental health consultation is a method for use between two professionals in respect to a lay client or a programme for such client.

2. The consultee's work problem must be defined by him as

being in the mental health area, relating to (*a*) mental or personality disorder of the client; (*b*) promotion of mental health of the client; and (*c*) interpersonal aspects of the work situation. It is assumed that the consultant has expert knowledge in these areas.

3. The consultant has no administrative responsibility for the consultee's work or professional responsibility for the outcome of the client's case. He is under no compulsion to modify the consultee's conduct of the case.

4. The consultee is under no compulsion to accept the consultant's ideas or suggestions.

5. The basic relationship between the two is coordinate, there being no built-in hierarchical authority which is expected to potentiate the influence of ideas and their easy adoption.

6. The coordinate relationship is fostered by the consultant being a member of another profession and a visitor.

7. Dependency is avoided as consultations are few, brief and intermittent.

8. Consultation is expected to continue indefinitely in that consultees are expected to encounter unusual work problems throughout their careers and increasing competence makes them more likely to recognise problems and demand more consultations.

9. A consultant has no predetermined body of information that he intends to impart to a particular consultee. He responds only to that segment placed before him, though other areas may be submitted at subsequent consultations.

10. The twin goals are to help the consultee improve his handling or understanding of the current difficulty and thus improve his capacity to master similar problems in future.

11. The aim is to improve the consultee's work and not his sense of well-being.

12. Consultation does not focus overtly on the consultee's personal problems and feelings. It respects his privacy. The consultant does not allow the discussion of personal and private material.

13. This does not mean that the consultant does not pay attention to the feelings of the consultee, but he deals with them in a special way such as the form in which the consultee has displaced them on to the client.

14. The consultant should be free to abandon the above rules if

he decides that the consultee's actions are endangering the client by overlooking the risk of suicide or serious mental breakdown. This breaks the coordinate relationship, but in favour of a higher goal.

15. Mental health consultation is not a new profession but merely a special way in which existing professionals operate.

Types of consultation: (1) client-centred; (2) consultee-centred; (3) programme-centred administrative; (4) consultee-centred administrative.

This movement is a rapidly developing one and has an obvious appeal to the politician. Its value to the community awaits proof.

What is meant by **family psychiatry?**

In certain instances it has been shown that an original patient referred was really a symptom of a family disturbance, and treatment directed at the patient alone would not solve the patient's or the family's problems. Because of this it is becoming more popular to get the whole family to come up for treatment and group discussion. Some ask the family to complete a questionnaire with moderately controversial, but homely, items regarding family life in adolescence and their culture. The papers are marked and returned and then the experimenter points out the differences and agreements. The family are then asked to reconsider the differences and explore the agreements. It has been recently used in hospitalised schizophrenics with encouraging results.

A deeper level of analytical interpretation may also be undertaken either when seeing the patient and members of the family together or separately. This has been used particularly by existential psychiatrists who see the schizophrenic patient as a symptom of the family's disturbance.

SECTION 16

CHILD PSYCHIATRY

List **Gesell's findings on the chronological achievements** *in infancy and childhood*

First three months. Control of eye muscles.

Second three months. Supports head, moves arms, reaches out.

Third three months. Controls trunk and hands; sits; grasps; manipulates objects.

Fourth three months. Controls legs, forefinger and thumb; pokes and plucks; stands.

Second year. Walks; runs; speaks; controls bowel and bladder; acquires sense of personal identity and possession.

Third year. Uses sentences; understands environment; complies with cultural demands.

Fourth year. Asks questions; perceives analogies; conceptualises and generalises; nearly self-dependent in home routines.

Fifth year. Mature motor control; hops and skips; loses infantile articulation; can narrate; prefers associative play; takes pride in clothes and accomplishment; self-assured and conforming citizen in his small world.

The child's growth extends through four major fields of behaviour: (1) motor; (2) adaptive; (3) language; (4) personal-social.

Summarise **Piaget's system of child development**

Piaget made a prolonged and intensive study of how children view the world around them and considers that intelligence develops through a sequence of progressively more complex patterns of action and thinking. Each step is regarded as a stage of development and each new type of behaviour or thinking is generalised to other aspects of reality though with some time lag.

Sensorimotor stage

Substage 1 (1st month). Reflex schemata, such as looking at light, attempting to grasp.

237

Substage 2 (approximately 1 to 4½ months). New schemata. The child fixates objects with eyes and follows moving ones; develops various hand movements; utters sounds and plays with his saliva.

Substage 3 (4½ to 8 or 9 months). Uses vision to direct hands to objects and to grasp them and he now is able to exercise some effects on objects, shaking pram and making toys dangle.

Substage 4 (8 or 9 to 11 or 12 months). Co-ordination of schemata in Substage 3.

Substage 5 (11 or 12 months to 18 months). More complex manipulations are evident and adaptive behaviour in problem solving is now apparent. Trial and error is commonly used with corresponding progress in construction of objective world and in imitation.

Substage 6 (18 months onwards). Solution of problems by invention of new means instead of by trial and error.

These stages then give way to the *pre-operational stage*:

(*a*) Symbolic and pre-conceptual stage. (1½ to 4 years).

(*b*) The intuitive stage (4 to 7 years).

These are followed by the *Concrete operational stage* (7 to 11 years) and *abstract operational thinking* (approximately 11 years onwards).

What is **ethology**?

Ethology is the study of behaviour of an animal in its normal environment. This has been extended to the field of child psychiatry as well as adult psychiatry. Conclusions are drawn which may be valid in the animal field but do not necessarily hold for human behaviour. It has been said that the ethologist has substituted for an anthropomorphic view of the rat a ratomorphic view of man.

Discuss the effect of **parent-child relationships** on child development

Much accent has been placed on frustration and conflict and their adverse effects in child rearing, but these need not be destructive in or of themselves. The child who is never frustrated, whose conflicts are resolved for him by eliminating or easing factors which prevent spontaneous expression and satisfaction of his desires, becomes well-adjusted only to an extremely artificial set of circumstances. At a later stage when socialisation is beyond the parents' control, as at school, he will lack the experience which would help him to know how to respond to each new situation. The child should not be seen as a *tabla rasa*, but may himself influence the parents' reaction. For example, difficulties with feeding may excite in the mother feelings of failure and guilt with associated anxiety and this in turn conditions her attitude to the child.

Interparental strife is commonly a disturbing influence on children, but there are other more subtle situations which may be even more disturbing.

Fathering

This is being given increasing accent and fathers are expected to show many of the maternal qualities in terms of fondling and playing the mother's role. This has been extended to encouraging him to be literally in at the birth by attending the labour ward. Many of the rules which govern parent-child relationships are the slaves of fashion and one sees them come and go, and it is very difficult to be sure whether the present fashion is the most helpful. It says much for the adaptability of the child that whatever the prevalent fashion he seems to emerge relatively unscathed.

This does not mean that parent-child relationships are of no importance, and certain factors have been stressed, such as *maternal over-protection* which may be a device for the denial of hate, particularly if the child was initially unwanted. It is alleged to be an expression of maternal guilt over unconscious hate and may take the form of an obsessional over-solicitude which extends into the many areas of contact between mother and child, such as feeding, nursing and dressing, and their prolongation beyond normal limits. Some of these mothers have their children sleep with them even in their teens, and make companions of them, thus depriving them of contemporary friendships and blunting their capacity to make easy contact with strangers.

Importance is attached to suckling and weaning, feeding and toilet training, and support for elaborating their influence on personality has come from anthropological studies, particularly those of Margaret Mead. *Familial influences* are being given equivalent accent to parental influences, and sentiments and conception of self and social imagery may well be qualities inculcated by the family and profoundly influence the character of the child. Among other familial influences are structural aspects of the family such as birth order and the number and sex of siblings. Very little reliable information has come from these studies to date. Neither do genetic aspects yield any conclusions except that constitution and environment are not as independent of each other as some investigators have maintained. In these fields it is easier to establish correlations than to interpret them.

What is a **normal child**?

A normal child gets along reasonably well with parents, siblings and friends, has few overt manifestations of behavioural disturbance, uses his apparent intellectual potential to a degree close to its estimate, and is contented for a reasonable proportion of the time. Shyness and boisterousness are normal qualities and should not be dressed up in words like 'schizoid' or 'hyperkinetic'. Frequently a normal child is paraded at a clinic in order to bring attention to parental instability and it is doubtful practice whether the child should be retained at the clinic in order to maintain contact with the parent. Arguments in favour of having a child attend a clinic in order to treat the parents should be overwhelming as it means divorcing a normal child from its normal surroundings.

Which features distinguish the **brain-damaged child**?

The syndrome usually incorporates hyperkinesis, distractability, short attention-span, labile mood, anti-social behaviour, anxiety and limited intelligence. The diagnosis rests on the following:

1. *History*, which may be of head injury, encephalitis, anoxia at birth, meningitis, or other trauma or inflammation of the brain and its coverings.

2. *Neurological signs and symptoms such as hemiplegia or hemianopia.*

3. *Special investigations.* (*a*) Physical, including air-encephalogram and electroencephalogram. There are wide variations in standards of normality at any one age, and making interpretations of these investigations can be extremely difficult. (*b*) Psycho-

logical tests, which include those for intelligence, measurement of perceptual anomalies and projection tests are notoriously unreliable. Most investigators who have studied the psychiatric sequelae of children with acute head injuries stress that these occur almost entirely in children with emotional disturbances before the injury and whose parents *and physicians* were anxious and over-protective. Children with behaviour disorders were also more prone to head injuries.

Describe **reactive behaviour disorders**

These may be a prolongation or reactivation of a normal reaction to a frightening experience and are seen particularly in childhood fears or phobic states, where an almost unrelated experience can trigger off an earlier reaction. A child who may have successfully resorted to tantrums to reach his objective, may use this pattern in less appropriate circumstances. Treatment is relatively simple and is mainly reassurance and a more steadying form of discipline.

List the commoner **neurotic behaviour disorders**

These represent deterioration of the reactive state described above. The common forms are:

1. Compulsive masturbation.
2. Tics.
3. Thumb-sucking.
4. Nail-biting.

What are **neurotic character disorders?**

These are said to be present when neurotic behaviour disorders are so ingrained that they play a major part in the formation of the child's character. Other people's attitudes, motives and conduct are distorted and as a result the neurotic behaviour engenders unfavourable environmental responses which in turn further engender neurotically defensive behaviour in a vicious cycle. They tend to be very resistant to psychotherapy.

Discuss the problem of **stammering in children**

This is synonymous with stuttering. It has been defined as an interruption in the normal rhythm of speech of such frequency and abnormality as to attract attention, interfere with communication, or cause distress to the stutterer or his audience. He knows precisely what he wishes to say but at the time is unable to say it easily because of an involuntary repetition, prolongation or cessation of sound. Two types are described; physiological or primary and pathological or secondary. In the second group boys are more commonly affected than girls and there is a positive correlation with low intelligence.

Emotional factors are important in determining and aggravating stammer and these require attention. Relaxation, speech therapy and hypnosis have all been tried with varying success.

Discuss the psychological problems of **sexual assaults on children**

Contrary to expectations, even promiscuous children are relatively unaffected by their experiences, and two categories have been described: the unaffected and the guilty. More commonly the person who is most upset is the parent. He or she may be convinced that this traumatic experience of the child must lead to neurotic behaviour.

Discuss the problem of **nocturnal enuresis** in children

The condition is said to exist when a child after the age of 3 frequently wets his bed. Organic factors have been traditionally regarded as important, such as spina bifida, but this must be a rare event. Evolutionary theories based on the maturation of the sleep pattern have been invoked and this could certainly explain it in infants. An infant wakes spontaneously only to be fed, and artificial waking for potting is paid for later by deeper sleep and enuresis. The enuretic child is more insecure and may seek refuge in hypersomnia, which does not permit the normal stimulus of a full bladder to waken the sleeper.

Treatment. This may initially be mainly directed towards breaking up faulty patterns of control which the parents have been trying, such as gestures, bribes, deprivation, punishment of all types, restriction of drinks which leads to a more concentrated urine with greater irritation, as well as frequent wakening at night. Successful treatment by psychotherapy is commonly reported, but much will depend on the interest the psychotherapist shows in the condition and his capacity to see the child's problem.

Remedies abound and include electric alarms which are set off by the contact of urine with a pad placed on the mattress, pituitary snuff, hypnotic suggestion and drugs such as ephedrine, amphetamine and more recently imipramine. With the latter, dosage is from 25 to 50 mg. each night for children from 5 to 7, to a maximum of 75 mg. over the age of 10. Treatment may have to be continued for two to three months.

What is **encopresis**?

This is involuntary defaecation not directly attributable to physical illness, and is diurnal rather than nocturnal. Precipitating factors may be starting school, the birth of another child or removal from home, and encopresis is regarded as an expression of hostility or retaliation for a fancied insult.

Describe the commoner **eating problems** of childhood

1. *Refusal of food*. This is a marked feature of Western civilisation and may be the resultant of two forces: (*a*) the urge for the parent to give and (*b*) the need for the child to deny. The three principal factors are: (1) culturally imposed mechanisation and over-regulation of feeding; (2) obsessive and coercive maternal over-protection; and (3) infantile response to maternal attitudes.

2. *Over-eating*. Food may be the only source of emotional satisfaction for the child, who, if it is insecure and unloved, may be unable to develop creative sources of satisfaction and takes to over-eating with resultant obesity. Treatment is directed to help the child to free himself from this form of dependence and become self-reliant and to make constructive use of his good physical and mental endowment.

3. *Aerophagy and rumination* (i.e. air-swallowing and the habit of bringing up food without nausea or retching). These can be a source of pleasure and therefore resistant to treatment. Rumination can be a severe problem because of the resultant dehydration and electrolyte loss.

4. *Anorexia nervosa*. In the child this problem is similar to that in the adolescent and may alternate with compulsive eating.

5. *Pica*. This is a craving for unnatural articles of food and is seen in pregnant women as well as in children.

Discuss the **psychosomatic disorders** *in childhood*

The commoner disorders are recurrent abdominal pain or, as it has been described, 'the little bellyacher', asthma, feeding and sphincter disturbances. Underlying all these is what has been known as 'the periodic syndrome' with recurrent abdominal, head or limb pains, vomiting and fever, which may occur singly as cyclic vomiting or a recurrent pyrexia or together. Diagnosis is based on negative evidence, such as the exclusion of the organic, and also by positive evidence which is the demonstration of emotional disturbance. A third factor in diagnosis is treatment itself which if directed at the emotional disturbance is more likely to succeed than if the symptoms are dealt with.

Discuss the **psychoses** *of childhood*

These are divided into organic and functional.

Organic. The commonest causes are encephalitis and meningitis, degenerative disorders such as Schilder's disease, cerebral tumours, hypertensive crises and chorea. Toxic states such as those due to lead and the ingestion of poisons such as belladonna, as well as febrile episodes may precipitate psychotic behaviour. More recently over-dosage of drugs such as amphetamine, thyroid or even alcohol are responsible for acute psychotic states.

Functional. These are traditionally divided into the manic-depressive and the schizophrenic varieties.

Manic-depressive. These are not as rare as was previously thought and a number of quite severe depressions present in childhood and pre-adolescence.

Schizophrenic. These differ from the adult in that the psychopathology with all its elaborations may not be the same. Language has not yet developed and life experiences are still limited and consequently delusional formations in childhood are relatively simple and their symbolisation is particularly naïve.

Aetiology. The biological concept has been advocated. A lag in maturation with disturbances in body image, identity and orientation to impersonal objects have been considered to be an essential factor in this concept. Evidence of this is the 'Whirling Test', which is based on the abnormal persistence of primitive postural and righting reflexes. The child is asked to close his eyes and stand with his arms extended and parallel. The child's head is then rotated as far as possible without discomfort. In a positive response the child turns his body in the direction of the rotation of the head as long as the pressure is applied.

Psycho-social factors have also been invoked. In a true functional state there is inadequacy of the child's physiological basis for receiving impressions, evaluating them, conceptualising and acting, and there is inadequacy of the child's psycho-social environment, i.e. the family, particularly in terms of its ability to enhance the child's efforts to structure his experiences, to give meaning to them, and to improve his adaptive efficiency.

Clinical features

1. Acute cases. Performance at school deteriorates, concentration is impaired and there may be an accompanying anxiety with the usual physical concomitants. Perplexity, restlessness, insomnia, bizarre hypochondriasis, in fact most of the features seen in the adolescent, including auditory hallucinations, may appear. Precipitating factors are again those found in the adolescent group, e.g. severe emotional upsets, operations and infections. The episode is usually short-lived and responds to treatment but it may drift into chronicity.

2. Insidious cases are difficult to recognise in the early stages. There is a gradual withdrawal and less tendency to engage in speech or communicate.

Many people equate childhood schizophrenia with childhood psychosis, much of which may be of organic origin. These childhood psychotic states usually meet the following criteria:

1. Gross and sustained impairment of emotional relationships with people.
2. Apparent unawareness of personal identity to a degree inappropriate to age.
3. Pathological preoccupation with particular objects.
4. Sustained resistance to change in environment.
5. Abnormal perceptual experience.
6. Acute, excessive and seemingly illogical anxiety.
7. Speech may have been lost or never acquired.

8. Distortion in motility patterns, for example hyperkinesis or immobility.

9. A background of serious retardation, with islets of normal or near normal intellectual function.

Schizophrenia, with the failure of ego-defences and subsequent ego-disintegration, is very rare in young children and generally does not manifest till puberty. The so-called 'psychotic' child to which the above nine points refer is more likely to be suffering from an organic cerebral disease than from schizophrenia. Many very young children are labelled schizophrenics because their behaviour is in part *analogous* to that found in schizophrenia but the analogy frequently ends there.

What is an **autistic child?**

This term derives from *primary infantile autism* first described by Kanner. Children in this stage make contact more easily with things than with people and they therefore do not learn to talk and may be considered mentally subnormal or aphasic. To establish a diagnosis there should be some evidence that the child is capable of ideation at a level higher than that of its capacity for speech. The aphasic child may be boisterous in company while the autistic child tends to be apathetic.

In Kanner's original cases, the parents of these children were of high intelligence, probably due to the fact that many of them were members of the staff of his university, and because of this it has been accepted in some quarters that mentally abnormal children of parents of high intelligence are necessarily autistic children. This of course need not be so, and this type of child may be born to parents who are not intelligent and many of the children of intelligent parents may be suffering from organic brain disorders producing the commoner forms of mental defect. The parents of these children being middle-class tend to be more articulate than the parents of mentally defective children and are able to influence the deployment of resources. Successes are claimed in the treatment of the autistic child but it is doubtful whether these are greater than would result in a series of mentally defective children who were favoured with similar attention. What was initially regarded as mainly a functional problem is becoming increasingly recognised as an organic one, in that post-mortem studies have shown some to be suffering from tuberous sclerosis and EEG studies have demonstrated that a number develop an epileptic record.

What part do **physical illness and handicaps** *play in child psychiatric disturbances?*

These are frequently quoted as causative of emotional disturbances, and parents are generally convinced of the relationship. The diabetic child who cannot tuck in to all the good things at a party; the cardiac child who is unable to join in at games; the polio victim who cannot walk or has to wear calipers, can all excite in the adult the capacity to project himself into the child's situation and 'understand' how the child must feel. Organ inferiority (see under Adlerian psychopathology) may explain the tendency for some children to over-compensate because of some physical defect, but it is the parents who are frequently more involved in these matters. They may over-protect and shelter and thus obstruct the normal processes which make for the child's independence. Some children tend to exploit this over-protection and react similarly in future situations.

What effect may **admission to hospital** *have on a child?*

Much attention has been given to this problem and it has been claimed that admission to hospital involving separation from the parents may give rise to anxiety and depression in the child, and much propaganda has been directed towards this. Obviously most children do not suffer, but a few who are vulnerable probably do. The tendency has been to apply a blanket remedy to the problem by insuring that all children have constant visiting in hospital by the parents although it must be admitted that frequently certain parents may be better excluded from visiting their child while in hospital, but this selectivity may be difficult to enforce. Children under 7 months do not exhibit this fretting behaviour, and it is generally agreed that in children over 5 years the need is not so great. On the other hand, a sick child tends to regress and chronological age may not indicate the emotional needs of the patient. The usual objections to having mothers visit their children or stay with the children in hospital, such as

I

nursing obstruction, cross-infection and frankly difficult mothers, are not serious obstacles and can usually be overcome with the advantage of the mother becoming an unpaid nurse.

What place may **school** play in the development of childhood disturbances?

Attending at school is a universal experience of children in societies which have compulsory education. It has become so much part of the normal background that one is apt to forget the upheaval it can represent in the lives of some children. Emotional factors may create learning-blocks in which the emotional problem is primary and the learning difficulties symptomatic, or there may be a primary learning difficulty caused by faulty brain functioning which directly interferes with the learning process, and it is important to distinguish the one from the other.

Primary learning difficulties are generally reflected in the child's capacity for speech or for writing, and the influence of cerebral dominance has been invoked to explain these. It is usually found that most learning difficulties may be overcome by a good relationship between the teacher and the child, even although an organic element may be suspected.

Discuss the problem of **adoption**

Adoption may be undertaken to fulfil the emotional needs of the adoptive parents. Subsequently, if the procedure is breaking down there may be considerable associated guilt feelings. The type of home, therefore, where the child goes is extremely important and its character or economic class will strongly influence the child's ultimate intellectual functioning whatever his genetic endowment and will also contribute to his stability. The following difficulties in adoption have been described:

1. Temporary adjustment problems, which can usually be overcome by counselling.
2. Threatened breakdown of placement and rejection of the infant. This calls for a complete re-appraisal of the adoption.
3. Telling the child. The child should be told at an early age that he is adopted and his questions answered frankly and sympathetically.

There is controversy as to whether the mother should see the child before she relinquishes it and some authorities advocate that she should and others that she should not. Most experienced workers advocate that the mother should not only see the child but breast feed it for the first month.

What is meant by **school phobia?**

It signifies a persistent refusal to attend school, the child remaining at home with full knowledge of his parents, as opposed to *truanting*, where the child usually absents himself from home and school. They tend to be more intelligent and of higher social class, work and behave better at school and are more timid, have been less frequently separated from their mothers in early childhood, have mothers who are over-protective, and have a higher incidence of family neurosis. Separation-anxiety rather than fear of school is the main problem and it has been suggested that they be called mother-philes rather than school-phobes. Many of these children receive home tuition, but when they are taken into hospital and treated as phobic anxiety of the adult kind, they usually respond to treatment and are able to continue with their normal education.

Discuss the problems of **children of psychotic parents**

Although theoretically this should be very disruptive of interpersonal relations and seriously affect the child's development, evidence of this has not been forthcoming. The evidence which has been reported is that if the child is under 2 no excessive neurotic features are shown, though these do increase but not significantly in the 3 to 5 age-group. A schizophrenic father is alleged to be less harmful than a schizophrenic mother, but even schizophrenic mothers can make excellent parents and rear normal children. When one considers the large incidence of schizophrenics in the population and the number who do have children, those children who seem adversely affected by their parentage must be very few indeed.

Discuss the **psychiatric problems of adolescence**

The majority of children seem to emerge from the adolescent phase unscathed, but for some it could be a stress situation and mental disturbances may result.

The stresses involved are those of *puberty*. This is a phase which can lead to difficulties, particularly in those who have an early or a late onset. Because of the associated secondary sexual characteristics, there is usually considerable focus of interest on these phenomena and their early or late emergence will be noted and remarked on. Failure to achieve an erection in a late-developing boy can accentuate his organ inferiority, and similarly, failure for the voice to break may result in suggestions of homosexuality. In the girl, early puberty may result in sexual precocity, for she may try to emulate the older girls and yet not have the intellectual and emotional maturity to handle the situations to which her conduct exposes her.

External stresses

These are usually of school and home. In the former there may be conflict between the increasing demands of the curriculum and the instinctive urges of puberty. Compulsive masturbation with associated expiation may lead to quite severe obsessional features and occasionally severe depression. The commoner problems in adolescence which one meets are obsessional states, phobic anxiety states including school phobia, anorexia nervosa, schizophrenic disorders and depressive states. Treatment for these is as for the adult.

Discuss **delinquency** in childhood

A child brought into court for having committed a delinquent act may be psychotic or neurotic, psychopathic or normal, intelligent or defective, physically healthy or manifesting behaviour chiefly derived from organic brain disease or an intolerable family or neighbourhood situation. The definition of delinquency, therefore, has legal limits, varies between different countries and states, depends on the efficiency of those forces responsible for detection and apprehension, and on the milieu of the child which may not inculcate that respect for law and order which society might wish.

The mentally normal is by far the commonest perpetrator of delinquent acts and even the finding of some mental abnormality may have no causal relationship. Conditions which have a causal relationship are (1) *the brain-damaged child*, (2) *reactive behaviour disorders*, leading to destruction of public property, (3) *the neurotic child* who reacts with aggression and hostility, (4) *the psychotic child*, rarely, (5) *the psychopathic child*, who does not differ markedly from the psychopathic adult, and (6) *the mentally subnormal child*.

Discuss **suicide and suicidal attempts in children**

Suicide and suicidal attempts are not as rare in childhood as has been previously considered. Among those who have attempted suicide the following causes have been defined: (1) anger at another which is internalised in the form of guilt and depression, (2) attempts to manipulate another to gain love and affection, or to punish another, (3) a signal of distress, (4) reactions to feelings of inner disintegration, as a response to hallucinatory commands, etc., and (5) a desire to join a dead relative.

What is **play therapy?**

A number of specialised toys which are said to be of fundamental importance in treatment have been devised. These include dolls that can be fed with bottles and which wet their 'nappies' and require changing. It is alleged that the child can identify more readily with these toys and act out its own problems in relation to feeding and excretion as well as sibling rivalries. A model house which can be used by a few children permits the child to take part in a group situation and act out those problems which may be related to the home and which would otherwise not be introduced into the clinic. Water and mud excite childhood reactions to excreta, and their manipulation may tap earlier memories and patterns of behaviour which had hitherto been dormant. The sand-tray with its numerous contents—houses, farms, cows, sheep, lambs, fences, soldiers, parental figures and other children—permits the creation of an infinite variety of situations and the display of attitudes to meaningful situations in the child's background. Questions and interpretations while the child is at play help in uncovering for the child some of those aspects which had been incompletely repressed and were leading to symptom formations. Painting and drawing have both therapeutic and diagnostic uses as they permit the child free expression, or indicate his inhibitions and restrictions. They can be interpreted and as they form part of the child's own creations. their content is likely to be significant.

Which forms of analytical psychotherapy are used?

This treatment has been established by the work of Anna Freud and Melanie Klein. Anna Freud considers that defence mechanisms in childhood differ from those in the adult and she describes the following: (1) denial in phantasy, (2) restriction of the ego, (3) identification with the aggressor, and (4) a form of altruism.

Melanie Klein believes that environmental factors are of much less importance than have previously been believed. She also stresses that the forerunners of the super-ego must be analysed and this really means going back in the child's life before the age of 2, and so lays the greatest emphasis on the child's aggressive drives. She centres her analysis around the phantasy life of the child as revealed in play. Interpretations are given directly and even the deepest interpretations may be given during the first meeting.

Discuss the treatment of the schizophrenic child

Such children usually relate better to objects than to people and such objects are exploited to lead the child to express its feelings. The following is an account of the treatment recommended by Chess:

1. One small segment of reality (such as a toy balloon) is employed as a basis for activity.

2. The physical nature of this object is explored. It is compared with other objects and the laws governing its behaviour under varying circumstances are examined.

3. In the course of play, these laws which are discovered are stated and restated.

4. Differences between the object and the young patient are established in terms of the play activity being carried on.

5. One after another, new activities are introduced. As each one enters the treatment situation the pattern of stating the laws which govern the activity is repeated, and the play is structured so as to necessitate examining and defining what is being done.

6. People are brought into the discussion and the significance of human wishes and desires are explained in the same kind of terms which are applied to objects.

7. Rules of behaviour are discussed and demonstrated. These include: what is expected of one in a given set of circumstances; what are good manners; what is meant by sharing; or by contrast, what hurts others or makes them uncomfortable. If necessary, an issue is made of forbidding or of demanding certain forms of behaviour.

What is the place of **behaviour therapy?**

The advantages which have been listed are: (1) non-verbal operation, (2) strict control of variables, (3) quantification of operations, (4) exclusion of 'clinician-variables', and (5) single-case studies.

These 'theoretical' considerations do not stand up to scrutiny in practice and, as in behaviour therapy with adults, it is the relationship between patient and therapist which really counts and this includes motivation and expectancy on both sides. To date there have been no significant reports which show that the new measures are any more successful than those used previously. When previous treatments have been successful their similarity to behaviour therapy has been stressed but only the committed would pursue this argument.

Discuss **maternal deprivation**

This concept has been given prominence by the work of Bowlby and has come to be regarded as a major aetiological factor in childhood psychiatric disorders. Rutter has pointed out much of the looseness in thinking associated with the term and that many of the alleged outcomes of maternal deprivation are not specifically tied to the mother and are not due to deprivation. He lists these specific conditions and adds his criticisms:

1. *Acute distress.* This is due in part to a disruption of the bonding process but the bonding is not necessarily with the mother. While deprivation is correct in describing this syndrome, the adjective 'maternal' may be misleading.

2. *Developmental retardation* is probably due to a lack of

stimulation rather than its loss and thus privation would be a more appropriate word than deprivation. Moreover, it is a lack of stimulation which matters and not mother's presence, so that 'experiential' is a better adjective than 'maternal'. It is the child's language environment which is important and the mere presence of an interested adult is not enough.

3. *Dwarfism.* Although Rutter claims that impaired food intake is the most important factor, other workers have found maternal deprivation equally important, so this factor is still debatable.

4. *Delinquency and antisocial disorders.* These are more likely to stem from distorted family relationships in general rather than from a distorted relationship with the mother.

5. *Affectionless psychopathy.* This is based on a failure to develop bonds or attachments in the first three years of life, leading to attention seeking, uninhibited indiscriminate friendliness and finally to a personality characterised by a lack of guilt and an inability to form lasting friendships. It is the bond formation that matters but this need not be with any particular person.

Write a short note on **battered babies**

Children with apparently unexplained or poorly explained injuries have for long been presenting at hospital casualty departments but it is in recent years that the size of the problem of the battered baby has been grasped by society. The condition should be suspected if a child sustains an unusual or severe injury and the parents have delayed in seeking advice or give unsatisfactory explanations of the 'accident'. A sequence of minor avoidable injuries or burns may occur. There may be a contrast between the attention to the child's clothes and cleanliness and its failure to gain weight.

The problem has recently been highlighted because of the failure of certain social service departments to take appropriate action under the Children & Young Persons' Act (1969) which permits the child or children to be taken into care 'if his proper development is being avoidably prevented or neglected or his health is being avoidably impaired or neglected or he is being ill-treated'. There is also a clause which permits preventive action if one child in a family has already died in a similar situation.

The concept of maternal deprivation is so strongly embedded in social work training that many social workers will not initiate removal of the child from the mother under any circumstances and the resulting tragedies have called into question social work training and the competence of social workers to deal with their statutory duties.

SECTION 17

MENTAL DEFICIENCY

What is **mental deficiency?**

Mental deficiency is not a disease, but a condition resulting from a variety of causes, inborn or acquired, whereby there is arrested mental development which is apparent from birth or from an early age. Although the terms 'idiot', 'imbecile' and 'feebleminded' (moron) are no longer official in Britain, it will still be necessary to define the different grades or severity of defect, if only on administrative grounds.

Idiots are so low-grade that they are unable to protect themselves from common physical dangers such as fire, heights or inedible matter, and have no language.

Imbeciles can learn to avoid these dangers and have a limited vocabulary which permits communication but are usually unable to learn to read or write or be trained to lead an independent existence.

Higher-grade defectives (*morons*) can benefit from formal education though they are frequently classed as educationally subnormal and have to attend a special school where their handicaps are given due attention, but they can learn to read and write and make the necessary social adjustments to maintain themselves independently in the community.

The Mental Health Act (1959) has only two categories, 'subnormal' and 'severely subnormal'.

What factors determine the **admission of a mental defective to an institution?**

Admission does not necessarily depend on degree of mental deficiency. Higher grades are frequently tempted into petty crime or prostitution and have not the ability to respond to ordinary corrective measures and may therefore be committed to institutions because the family or society are unable to control their behaviour. Lower grade defectives, on the other hand, may be much more amenable to social restraint and can reside at home.

256

There is a class bias towards institutional care in that middle-class families tend to seek such care more often than lower-class families. Rural areas do not offer the same temptations to petty crime that are met in the city and therefore the prevalence of these disorders would appear to be less in these areas. Once a rural area becomes urbanised, the incidence of mental defectives requiring institutional care begins to rise.

Discuss the role of **genetics** in mental deficiency (general factors)

There is some evidence that dullness tends to beget dullness, but there are also signs that stocks can mend and it is now not unknown for a person born of defective parents in an institution to have these same parents out on licence under his or her care. Social factors may influence mental development and a secure and happy home may help a child to a higher level of performance on intelligence tests than one who is deprived, so what is really a social factor may be attributed to genetic factors.

Define **mental defect**

No satisfactory definition exists, but certain criteria are regarded as useful.

1. *Social incompetence* based on lack of prudence, economic dependence, and failure in citizenship.

2. *Mental subnormality* which leads to No. 1 for reasons other than from physical handicap or socio-economic disadvantage.

3. *Developmental retardation* which is not due to deterioration but to arrest.

4. *A condition obtaining at maturity* which is therefore incurable or irremediable other than by habit-training.

5. *Of constitutional origin* either from hereditary lack of potential or through trauma, disease or deprivation, making normal adult status unlikely.

What is meant by the **I.Q. (intelligence quotient)**?

This is measured by a test which has both validity and reliability.

Validity is the degree to which a test measures what it claims to measure.

Reliability is the degree to which a test measures the same thing, the same way, at different times.

I.Q. is not a constant factor because this can vary according to errors in measurement, test familiarity, incorrect testing based on the experience of the tester, testing in a disturbing situation, too short a test, and variations in the rate of intellectual growth.

What is meant by **mental age?**

This term was frequently used instead of I.Q. but is now losing favour because of some of its failings, such as (a) lack of equality between age growth and mental growth, (b) lack of meaning of the term in adults, (c) the changes in the processes measured at different ages, and (d) the differences of meaning of the same mental age at different chronological ages.

Discuss **environmental factors** in mental deficiency

These are becoming increasingly recognised, especially in slum areas of cities. Deprived communities may produce a higher degree of children who are apparently mental defective. This has been shown in Negro scores in the U.S. Army which were below those scored by White recruits, but on the other hand Negro recruits from some of the Northern States were superior to White recruits from the Southern States. Children from foster homes do worse in tests than those from secure families, and imbecile children with no evidence of organic impairment tend to have exceptionally adverse homes which has been ascribed to 'pathological mothering'. This does not mean that an adverse environmental condition in itself can produce an imbecile grade, but that it makes a substantial contribution.

What is meant by **dermatoglyphics?**

These are dermal ridge arrangements in the hands and soles of feet and have been used to discriminate between monozygotic and dizygotic twins, and between mongols and normals. The classical ridge is the single transverse palmar (simian) crease which is more frequently found in children with congenital conditions and mental deficiency. It is now regarded as an indicator of impaired foetal growth very early in embryonic life which may manifest either as mental deficiency or other evidence of mal-development.

Discuss the **dominant defects** *associated with mental deficiency*

Dominant defects have the following three criteria:

(*a*) Sharp distinction between affected and unaffected members of the family.
(*b*) Every affected person has an affected parent.
(*c*) Approximately one half of the children will be affected in every sibship where there is an affected parent.

The following conditions are due to dominant defects.

Tuberous sclerosis

The classical triad of this condition was epilepsy, mental deficiency and adenoma sebaceum, giving rise to the term *epiloia*. It does not invariably present with this classical triad and lesions may appear in many places, such as:

(a) *Skin*. Adenoma sebaceum—a nodular rash of the characteristic butterfly spread on nose and cheeks, though it may also be on the forehead and chin; peau chagrin (Shagreen patch) on the lumbar region which does not appear till puberty; subungual (fingers and toes) fibromata and in rare instances it can be associated with neurofibromatosis.
(b) *Visceral tumours* in kidney and heart, but also in lung as well as brain.
(c) *Brain*. Mainly periventricular tumours which may calcify and are easily seen on X-ray. These may become malignant and resemble a rapidly growing glioblastoma.
(d) *Eye*. Grey-yellow-white plaques (phakomata) of varying size are seen on the retina in about half the cases.

Mental changes. Severe degrees of defect are the rule, but it may sometimes occur with high-grade defect or normal intelligence.

Epilepsy. This can be very severe and difficult to control and some of the psychotic features noted may be due to temporal lobe lesions.

Neurofibromatosis

Mental defect is not severe and occurs in only about 30 per cent of cases.

Rud's syndrome

Congenital ichthyosis with epilepsy and mental deficiency and occasionally spasticity.

Haemangiomatosis

(a) *Sturge-Weber syndrome.* This shows cutaneous facial angiomatosis (always extending above the palpebral fissure); gyriform calcification (radiographically apparent after the age of 2 years) underlying an area of leptomeningeal angiomatosis which is unilateral and usually confined to the posterior half of the brain; mental deficiency and epilepsy; buphthalmos and hemiparesis.

(b) *Von Hippel-Lindau.* Here the angioma involves the retina and cerebellum.

Cranio-facial dysostosis

The mental defect may be due either to the mechanical effect of skull change or to independent brain lesion.

Acrocephaly (oxycephaly)

An abnormally high or pointed head found in a variety of syndromes.

(a) *Crouzon.* Exophthalmos with small orbits and narrow optic foramina. Increased intracranial pressure may result.

(b) *Apert.* Ocular hypertelorism (wide separation of the eyes) and syndactyly.

Marfan's syndrome (dystrophia mesodermalis)

This is a generalised disorder of connective tissue characterised by very long extremities, including fingers and toes (arachnodactyly or spidery fingers). Ectopia of lenses, congenital heart defect and aneurysm of the aorta may also be present. Mental retardation is common but may not be severe.

Long fingers may be normal, but in Marfan's syndrome they can be defined by using a 'metacarpal index', arrived at as follows: the lengths of the right second, third, fourth and fifth metacarpals as seen on a radiograph are measured and the breadth of each metacarpal at its exact midpoint is also measured. A figure for each metacarpal is obtained by dividing the length by the breadth and the average of the four is taken. The normal range is said to be from 5·4 to 7·9 whereas in Marfan's syndrome it is 8·4 to 10·4. An index greater than 8·4 is therefore diagnostic of arachnodactyly.

Sjögren's syndrome (1950)

Hereditary congenital spino-cerebellar ataxia accompanied by congenital cataract and oligophrenia.

How do **recessive defects** *contribute to mental deficiency?*

The following criteria are cited:

1. Affected and unaffected persons in the same family can be sharply distinguished.
2. Parents and all immediate ancestors are unaffected.
3. Father and mother are blood relations more frequently than expected.
4. More than one offspring is likely to be affected.
5. Occasionally cases occur in collateral branches of the same family.

Many of these conditions are associated with disorders of amino-acid transport which are becoming increasingly recognised with paper chromatographic separation. Those associated with mental deficiency are:

Phenylketonuria (Phenylpyruvic amentia)

This was described initially by Fölling in 1934. The defect in protein metabolism is an inability to metabolise phenylalanine to tyrosine. Instead it is de-aminated into phenylpyruvic acid which with the phenylalanine and phenylacetic acid are excreted in the urine. Phenylpyruvic acid in an acid medium gives a green reaction to ferric chloride with subsequent colour fade, and this is used as a diagnostic test.

· *Clinical features.* Most are low grade, but imbecile and feeble-minded cases occur; it is rare in people of high intelligence. Patients are frequently undersized with blonde or reddish-brown hair, reduced head size and widely spaced incisors. Some suffer from a severe and stubborn chronic eczema and occasionally epileptic attacks. Healthy relatives show a normal phenylalanine level which rises and remains high after its ingestion. The incidence in mental deficiency institutions is less than 1 per cent.

Pathology. There is demyelinisation of the optic, cortico-ponto-cerebellar and corticospinal systems, an increase of astrocytes and microglia and a decrease in Purkinje cells. The substantia nigra and locus coeruleus of the brain are deficient in pigment and there is a lack of tyrosine and methionine in the adrenals.

Treatment. A phenylalanine-free diet has been said to cure the condition, but initial enthusiastic reports are now being criticised. Some do badly with the diet and develop a rash and fail to gain weight, yet with the addition of milk containing phenylalanine a dramatic recovery can result.

Maple syrup urine disease

This is characterised by increased excretion of the branched chain amino acids, leucine, isoleucine and valine in the urine with the smell of maple syrup, as well as high levels in the plasma. The infant fails to thrive, vomits and shows signs of severe cerebral degeneration. It is usually rapidly fatal and treatment is to date ineffective.

Hartnup disease

This is generalised amino-aciduria of renal origin called after the family in which it was first described. All amino acids except proline, hydroxyproline, methionine and arginine are increased in the urine to 5 to 15 times normal while the plasma amino acids are 30 per cent lower than normal. The primary defect is a decreased absorption of tryptophan from the jejunum and diminished reabsorption of tryptophan and other amino acids by the proximal renal tubule. Urinary excretion of indoxyl sulphate (indican) and indolacetic acid is invariably increased and can be further augmented by injection of tryptophan.

Symptoms are variable and may include a pellagra-like rash, cerebellar ataxia, diplopia, nystagmus and slow mental deterioration. Treatment by oral nicotinamide improves most symptoms except the mental ones.

Fructose intolerance

This is associated with slight mental and physical retardation and attacks of vomiting and unconsciousness can be precipitated by certain sweet foods containing fructose. A test dose confirms the diagnosis.

Arginnio-succinuria

Large quantities of arginnio-succinic acid are excreted in the urine (2 to 5 grammes in 24 hours). This acid is an intermediate in the ornithine-urea cycle and the disease is characterised by severe mental defect and occasionally fits. The hair is unusually friable. There is no treatment to date.

What other **metabolic disorders** are associated with mental deficiency?

1. Citrullinuria.

2. Hyperuricaemia. These patients in addition show cerebral palsy, choreo-athetosis and self-biting.

3. Cystathioninuria. The urine chromatogram shows peaks identical with *l*-cystathionine with excretion of 960 to 1300 mg./day and a C.S.F. content of 0·21 mg. per 100 ml. Clinical features are acromegaly; bilateral grooves in the scalp of the lateral occiput; small ears with pre-auricular fistulae on the left; bilateral conductive deafness; enlarged tongue; thyroid gland enlarged ×2; liver and spleen palpable; poor score on testing (Wechsler); poor concentration and judgment.

4. The lipoidoses. These are diseases involving the accumulation of lipids. Those generally associated with mental defect are:

Amaurotic family idiocy (Tay-Sachs). Originally described in the children of Jews of Eastern European descent, but also found in children of different origin. It starts in infancy and rapidly deteriorates, with death in about two years and is manifest by failure to develop mentally with blindness, paralysis and a characteristic cherry-red spot on the macula, though at times it can be grey. Other types are:

(*a*) Late infantile. There is no macular spot.
(*b*) Juvenile. Visual disturbance appears first at about 5 to 8 years.

Gargoylism (Hurler's syndrome). The bones of head and face are affected with protruding forehead and broad nose and jaw—hence the term gargoylism. There are other skeletal deformities, particularly of phalanges and metacarpals, and the abdomen may be protuberant with umbilical hernia. There are two forms, one in males, which is sex-linked with clear corneas and deafness, the other with cloudy corneas with autosomal recessive transmission. It is said to be due to a disorder of polysaccharide metabolism with lipid deposit in the brain with ballooning of the cell bodies—a change similar to that found in amaurotic family idiocy.

Laurence-Moon-Biedl syndrome

This starts in early life and is associated with retinitis pigmentosa causing a variety of visual defects; polydactyly of hands and/or feet; mental defect; obesity of the hypopituitary type; hypogenitalism; and diabetes insipidus.

Hepato-lenticular degeneration (Wilson's disease)

It is associated with a defect in copper metabolism in which the bound copper is decreased because of the defective synthesis of ceruloplasmin, a protein used in binding copper (90 per cent in the blood). As a result the unbound copper is increased and interferes with oxidation enzymes which may lead to lesions in brain and liver. Blood copper is low (20 to 50 mg. per cent) and urinary copper is high ($\times 100$). The liver is cirrhotic and there is degeneration of the lentiform nucleus and cerebral cortex with copper in liver, brain and cornea. It usually occurs in adolescence and presents with chorea-athetosis, mental deterioration and occasionally behaviour disorders. A typical feature is the Kayser-Fleischer ring—a brown copper deposit seen in the cornea. Treatment is to get rid of the copper with the anti-metallic drugs—Versene, BAL and penicillamine.

Give an account of mongolism

The name was derived because of a fancied resemblance in the eyes of these patients which are almond-shaped with epicanthic folds. Other than this single feature there is absolutely nothing to identify the condition with the Mongolian race. In order not to offend racial susceptibilities the term Down's syndrome is being used.

Aetiology

Genetic factors.   Several varieties are recognised.

1. **Trisomy-21 (autosomal trisomy-G).**   The extra chromo-some is a small acrocentric numbered 21.   Affected individuals are trisomic for this chromosome and the total complement is 47 instead of 46 chromosomes.   It has been suggested that chromo-some-21 carries loci for the ABO blood groups, leucocytic alkaline phosphatase and galactose-1-phosphate uridyl transferase. The extra chromosome had been previously regarded as a 21 because it bore a 'satellite' which is a minute speck of chromatic material at the end of the chromosome and separated from the body by a poorly staining zone.   These satellites are found only on acrocentric chromosomes and are found regularly on two of the G group though not always on the 21 chromosome, which can now be more clearly distinguished from 22 by the fluorescent banding technique.

Although the parents of mongols do not have detectable chromosomal abnormalities, they are reputed to have an increased incidence of taste abnormalities, such as insensitivity to quinine and some thiourea type compounds.   The much greater incidence in older mothers suggests that the abnormality may result from non-disjunction during meiosis of the oocyte when there is incorrect segregation of migration of the chromosomes into the daughter cells of that division.

It accounts for about 85 per cent of cases of Down's syndrome and the overall incidence is 1:700 live births with a marked variability according to maternal age; in early child-bearing years the incidence is 1:2000 live births, but it rises to 1:50 in mothers over 40 years.

2. **Translocations.**   These are generally found in young mothers and are therefore not related to increasing maternal age. The patient has 46 chromosomes, but one is larger and atypical due to an extra chromosome-21 becoming attached to either a member of the D (13–15) or the G (21–22) groups.   It is usually transmitted through the mother but G:G (21:21 or 21:22) translocation often stems from the father with a mean paternal age of 42·5 years, which is 10·8 years in excess of the overall mean paternal age.   Translocation mongols have a high incidence of neck webbing.

Theoretically, the chance is 1:3 that a mother with a D/G translocation will have a mongoloid child but the actual risk is lower (about 1:5). If the father carries the D/G translocation, the chance of having a mongoloid child is only 1:20. In extremely rare instances the translocation involves both 21-chromosomes of the G group, which join to form an isochromosome, and the chance of a mongoloid child is 100 per cent. Some translocations, usually of the D/G type, occur spontaneously in the child of genotypically normal parents. In this rare event the chance of a mongoloid sibling is the same as for the more common sporadic trisomy form.

3. **Mosaics.** As a result of non-disjunction in the fertilised zygote a few cases have two cell lines, one normal and one with 47 chromosomes. The relative proportion of each cell line is very variable from individual to individual. They tend to have a few of the typical characteristics of mongols, and are usually more intelligent with less pronounced physical stigmata and different dermatoglyphics.

4. **Double Trisomics.** These patients have 48 chromosomes (usually XXY or XXX together with trisomy 21).

Other factors for which there is some evidence in aetiology are:

1. Maternal age at birth.
2. The state of the uterine mucosa.
3. Endocrine disturbances.
4. Infective hepatitis.

Incidence. It is the commonest condition in mental defective institutions and the risk is about 1 per 1000 live births.

Clinical features. These are numerous and only several need be present to establish a diagnosis. The patient is short, and exhibits the following features: *Skull,* small and brachycephalic with flattened occiput. Fontanelles close late. *Eyes,* palpebral fissures are slanting and narrow with epicanthic folds. Strabismus, myopia and cataract are common and the iris shows white or light yellow spots at regular intervals (*Brushfield* spots) which are considered the most reliable guide to the diagnosis in the newborn. As the iris darkens with age, they disappear or become small whitish stripes. Conjunctivitis and blepharitis frequently occur. *Teeth* are irregular and small and there is a congenital absence of some permanent teeth, particularly the maxillary and mandibular lateral incisors and the second bicuspids. *Ears* are small, rounded and stick out. *Palate* is flat at the sides and elevated in the middle and has been called the omega (Ω) palate. *Tongue* is large and fissured (scrotal) and often protrudes. *Nose* is short. *Extremities* are short, particularly the hands. *Skin* is rough and dry. *Hands* show the little finger bent inwards with a reduction in size of its middle phalanx and the palms show a single transverse crease at the base of the four fingers. *Feet* show a cleft between the big and little toes. *Hair* is scanty and may be absent in the axillae while alopecia is common; *hypogenitalism*. *Heart* malformations are common and many die at birth because of them. These are usually septal defects (atrial or ventricular), but ostium atrio-ventriculare commune has been described as the most common severe malformation and it is alleged that this is almost never encountered in non-mongols. *Muscles* are hypotonic. *Joints* are lax; susceptibility to *respiratory infection*; *epilepsy* is *very rare*.

Intelligence. The physical signs are usually but not invariably associated with mental defect of the imbecile grade, but idiocy and feeblemindedness can also occur.

Personality. They are generally cheerful and friendly and good mimics, but naturally these features are not universal.

Treatment. There is no specific measure available and most are ineducable, though the impression is gained that the intelligence level is rising and that a number will qualify for education in special schools. Because of their docile and affectionate natures, many parents are reluctant to commit them to institutions and they tend to form a large part of the population of Occupational Centres. There they can be trained to a high level of social competence but are usually unable to lead an independent existence. Expectation of life was formerly not high, but the picture has changed with the advent of antibiotics in the treatment of respiratory infections and no doubt the cardiac surgeon will eventually make his contribution.

What is the place of amniocentesis in diagnosis and genetic counselling?

Amniotic cell culture has a high success rate in the prenatal diagnosis of Down's syndrome. It involves withdrawing 10–20 ml.

of amniotic fluid between the 14th and 16th weeks of gestation, using the trans-abdominal approach. In familial cases of trans-location Down's syndrome each subsequent pregnancy should be monitored. Foetal chromosomes can be readily distinguished in the cultured amniotic fluid cells and diagnosis can usually be made. If the foetus has 46 chromosomes and among them the trans-location chromosome, the parents should be told that their child will have Down's syndrome so that they may consider therapeutic abortion. If in subsequent pregnancies there are normal preg-nancies then the pregnancy should not be terminated. The whole question of foetal diagnosis with a view to abortion of a handi-capped foetus is a very controversial one and recent developments are making it more difficult.

Other genetic disorders detectable in cultured amniotic fluid cells

(1) Maple syrup urine disease; (2) Homocystinuria; (3) Cyst-athioninuria; (4) Galactosaemia; (5) Glycogen storage disease (Types I, II, III and IV); (6) Lesch-Nyhan syndrome (hereditary hyperuricaemia); (7) Lysosomal acid phosphatase deficiency; (8) Tay-Sachs disease; (9) Refsum's disease; (10) Muco-poly-saccharidoses (Hurler's and Hunter's syndromes and other variants); (11) Hypervalinaemia.

What is the **cri du chat syndrome?**

The patients have a curious weak mewing cry which appears to be due to weakness and underdevelopment of the upper part of the larynx, with a small, soft and very mobile epiglottis. Mental deficiency is usually more severe than in mongols, but much less so than in the other well-established autosomal defects.

The face is characteristically round with wide-set eyes that have an anti-mongoloid slant, low-set ears and small lower jaw with microcephaly. Transverse-palmar creases are common and occasionally there is a congenital heart lesion such as a patent ductus arteriosus.

The chromosome abnormality is a simple deletion of the short arm of one of the four 4 to 5 chromosomes. Usually only one member of the family is affected.

What is **embryopathy?** *and describe some examples*

Embryopathy is damage to the child by a variety of agents before birth.

Genetic microcephaly

This can be due to causes other than the recessive gene, for it is found after X-ray overdosage and rubella in the first months of pregnancy, and is usually divided into a primary genetic form and a secondary exogenous form. The face is characteristic, being bird-like or Aztec with a low cephalic index (breadth-length). The majority are imbecile.

Rubella

Following German measles in the mother during gestation, children may be born with congenital cataracts, but mental deficiency also occurs, and may be accompanied by congenital heart defects, microcephaly, partial or total nerve deafness with occasionally deaf-mutism. The earlier the infection the greater the incidence of congenital disorders, and it also depends on the type of epidemic as some produce a greater crop of defects than others.

Syphilis

Infection is usually by the mother through the placental circulation. Early infection produces foetal death and abortion, while later, diffuse or localised meningovascular lesions result. Early pregnancies are more vulnerable than later ones and a history of miscarriages is a frequent precursor to the birth of a syphilitic child. The disease is not nearly so common because of antibiotics and more effective ante-natal care reducing maternal syphilis. The dullness associated with the condition may be an expression of familial dullness rather than due to the infection. A rare type is juvenile general paralysis which shows rapid mental deterioration with serological and pathological changes similar to those in the adult. Hydrocephalus is usually mild.

Toxoplasmosis

The pathogen is a protozoon, toxoplasma, which has been found in birds, rodents, dogs and cats and is transmitted to the foetus by the infected mother, but it can also be acquired in infancy and the young or embryonic brain is particularly vulnerable.

Clinical features are mental defect, chorio-retinopathy, cerebral calcification, hydro- or microcephaly and epilepsy. The parasites may be found in the C.S.F. and serological tests are positive.

Pathology. Cystic granulomatous encephalitis with ventricular dilatation and cortical atrophy. The brain parenchyma shows areas of necrosis filled with phagocytic gitter cells with gliotic and granulomatous scars surrounding. The lesions are near the ventricles and in the cortêx, and a 'Swiss cheese pattern' is seen on microscopic examination. Although the condition is considered rare, it is likely to be more frequently reported now that it is generally recognised.

Broad thumbs and toes and facial abnormalities

This is a relatively new syndrome where children have the above abnormalities as well as beaked noses. Consistent dermatoglyphic patterns lend support to the new syndrome. Aetiological factors have not yet been defined.

Erythroblastosis foetalis (kernicterus; haemolytic disease of the newborn)

If blood from a rhesus monkey is injected into a rabbit, the rabbit's serum will then agglutinate over 80 per cent of the white population and these people are called Rh-positive, while approximately 15 per cent would not agglutinate and are called Rh-negative; this Rh factor is said to be a complex of antigens inherited as a Mendelian dominant.

In certain cases only an Rh-negative mother whose husband is Rh-positive may produce an Rh-positive foetus and develop the anti-Rh agglutinins in her blood during pregnancy and these enter the foetal blood stream through the placenta. If the mother has been previously exposed to Rh-positive blood either by pregnancy or blood transfusion, the stage is set for a mass reaction with severe haemolytic disease in the newborn child, who may be born dead or rapidly succumb. Should the child survive, severe jaundice develops, usually before 36 hours. The central nervous system may be permanently damaged, the basal ganglia being particularly vulnerable, hence the name kernicterus (nuclear jaundice).

Pathology. The lentiform nuclei, thalamus, hypothalamus and *cornu Ammonis* are yellow and the *corpora luysii* especially so. The pyramidal tracts are spared.

Clinically the picture is variable and may be one of general athetosis, persistent spasticity, ataxic or atonic diplegia. Nuclear deafness and speech defects have been described, but the commonest feature is mental defect.

Treatment. The early recognition of the possibility of the disease developing has resulted in birth control, the parents hazarding one child, but perhaps not a second. Exchange transfusions as soon as the condition develops have also reduced the incidence and the number of cases of kernicterus entering institutions is dwindling.

Drugs

The world-wide aftermath following the use of thalidomide by pregnant women has spot-lighted the serious risks of producing deformed and defective children by prescribing new drugs to expectant mothers. No doubt, drugs will be blamed for producing all these tragedies, some of which may well have been caused by other embryopathic agents, but it cannot be too strongly emphasised that drugs which are prescribed to such vulnerable patients should be absolutely essential and have no tainting of toxicity. Substitutes for well-tried, efficient and *safe* preparations should have overwhelming advantages to be given a trial.

What are the mental sequelae of **birth trauma?**

Pre-natal

These can be due to a variety of causes such as prematurity, Caesarian section, high forceps delivery and a variety of causes of anoxia, such as anaesthesia, twisted umbilical cord and protracted labour. The range of mental defect is great and is not proportionate to the physical handicap. Epilepsy is a frequent concomitant.

Post-natal

Head injuries are frequently quoted by parents of children with mental defect. Head injuries are extremely common in all children and there are a number of instances reported where serious damage and even death has resulted from slight injuries. The sequel will depend on the site and severity of the damage, but before attributing the defect to the post-natal trauma there should be a history of normal development till the time of the accident.

What are the mental sequelae of **poisoning** in children?

The commonest poison to which children are exposed is lead, which is especially dangerous as it has a particular affinity for brain tissue. The common sources are lead toy soldiers, lead paint which can be scraped off doors and walls, from brightly painted cribs and nipple shields, and fumes from burning lead-lined batteries. In addition to paralysis, anaemia and encephalo-pathy, there may be serious impairment of mental development. It is essential to estimate blood levels, the normal being 36 mg./100 ml. Two clinical types are described, acute and chronic, though the latter may give rise to acute episodes. Treatment is with the anti-heavy metal group, such as BAL, versene and calcium di-iodine-ethylene diamine (Ca EDTA). Penicillamine has been favoured as it can be given by mouth. Prophylaxis should be directed at the exclusion of lead from paints where children are housed, and from their toys.

What are the mental sequelae of **infections**?

Meningitis is a common condition which can be caused by a variety of agents but is primarily meningococcal or tubercular, though it is becoming less common as a cause of mental defect with the success of antibiotics.

Encephalitis is probably still the commonest cause, and can be mild or severe, though the subsequent development of mental defect may be unrelated to the severity of the infection. A variety of types may contribute, and one should enquire about a history of measles, mumps, whooping-cough, chickenpox, scarlet fever, rheumatic fever, vaccination against smallpox, and in patients from appropriate backgrounds, typhus, Rocky Mountain spotted fever, rabies, psittacosis, equine, St. Louis and Japanese encephalitis.

Clinical features. These are: motor disturbance of an extra-pyramidal nature; intellectual defect with learning difficulty; personality disturbance associated with hyperkinesis and defici-encies in social orientation; impulse disorders which may be quite violent leading to suicide and even homicide.

Although the causes are many, the clinical picture is fairly constant and does not give much indication of the responsible agent. Neurological signs and severe mental defect are more prevalent when the infection occurred in infancy, while behaviour disturbance with mild mental defect predominates in later infections.

Pathology. Macroscopically, there is depigmentation of the substantia nigra of the midbrain, with fibrous gliosis which extends to the periventricular grey matter of the midbrain and diencephalon. The histological reaction will depend on the stage of the disease; in the early stage there is an inflammatory reaction with perivascular cuffing, and in the later stages there is an 'outfall' of nerve cells in the substantia nigra, which is regarded as the most characteristic lesion.

Treatment is mainly education and rehabilitation and some remarkable successes can be achieved.

Discuss the role of **endocrine factors** in mental deficiency?

Many defectives show features of endocrine dysplasia, but only in a few instances are these causally related and the mechanism is obscure.

Hypothyroidism

The thyroid through its influence on cardiac output, enzymatic processes in the brain, water metabolism and oxygen utilisation, can interfere with cerebral function, but its exact method of action is still unknown.

Cretinism

This is due to lack of function of the thyroid in the newborn. It is not a single entity and a variety of types have been described. The commonest one is *endocrine cretinism* which is found in mountainous and hilly regions which are remote from the sea where there is a deficiency of iodine in the diet. The classical picture is that of dwarfism; dry skin; myxoedema; low B.M.R.; delayed carpal development; hypothermia; constipation; and severe mental defect which can amount to idiocy. Regions affected are Switzerland, Rocky Mountains and Derbyshire, and the condition has been largely controlled by the prophylactic introduction of iodine to the diet by adding it to the salt in the proportion of 5 mg. of Pot. Iod. to 1 kg. salt. When the condition has developed treatment is with a daily dose of thyroid 60 mg. for the first year of life, increasing to 120 to 200 mg. in later childhood.

Discuss the **social aspects of** *mental deficiency*

The main developments are those which provide alternative forms of treatment outside the institution, and also more rapid discharge of patients. Informal admission has helped to ease the burden of the mental defective in the community for it is now possible for parents with a defective child to get away for a holiday or have several weeks' rest while the child is cared for in the institution. In this way one hospital bed can serve up to 12 patients while previously it would have been blocked by one. *Occupation Centres* in urban areas where access is easy provide an adequate alternative for a large number of low-grade patients. Local authorities who have a financial obligation for the supervision and after-care of mental defectives have been quick to see the advantages of procuring employment for higher grade patients, especially in the Parks and Salvage Departments. There they can work under supervision and are cushioned against the fluctuations of the labour market.

In the institutions themselves there has been a change in the types of jobs the patients are trained to do. From the usual crafts such as bootmaking and repairing, tailoring, brush-making, rug-making, portering, gardening and horticulture, training is now geared for fitting the patient for employment in industry, and industrial centres are now a feature in most mental deficiency hospitals.

Social training. This has been given greater emphasis because it is now recognised that much of the breakdown of the defective in the community is not so much his lack of industrial skill but his lack of social adaptation. It is therefore important that while in an institution he should be encouraged by certain incentives in terms of money and privileges and that the whole programme should be as near that as the work life in the community. Because of this patients clock in; tea breaks are organised; overalls are worn; and factory hygiene is practised.

A lower-grade patient is trained to recognise essential items, such as traffic signals, and words like 'canteen', 'toilet', 'men', 'women', 'cloaks' rather than receive formal education in reading and writing.

What factors should be taken into consideration in the vocational and social **rehabilitation** *of the feebleminded?*

1. Subnormal intelligence.
2. Educational backwardness regardless of I.Q.
3. Lack of general knowledge regardless of I.Q.
4. Background of adverse experiences.
5. Emotional hunger.
6. Ambivalence to authority.

This list is very useful for it indicates the fields in which breakdown has arisen or is likely to occur and to what ends rehabilitation and remedial measures should be directed. Previously, consideration of the problem of mental deficiency was largely in terms of supervision and care which led to answers emphasising the defectives' disabilities. An approach based on the above considerations does not consider the hospital to be the only or the best solution to the problem and emphasises the overcoming of these disabilities which may turn out to be less formidable than was originally thought.

Discuss the problems in dealing with the **parents of mental defectives**

Parents may wish to deny the existence of the handicap yet have a desire to know the truth, and it is this ambivalence which can prove very difficult in management and treatment. Although the condition may be an obvious one and lend itself to a 'spot-diagnosis', such as mongolism, tuberous sclerosis or some other form of brain damage, it is important to undertake a thorough examination for it is a sound medical principle, and justice must also appear to be done. If the result of the examination, which should include a full history from the parents, is unequivocal, then the parents should be told. It is much kinder to settle their doubts than to protect oneself with a vague statement and have them lead the child round to a whole series of doctors, none of whom is prepared to commit himself to a diagnosis, which in fact presents no clinical difficulties.

To answer their relevant questions will demand a thorough knowledge of their domestic and financial circumstances, their plans for more children and the effect of the patient on the sibs. This is frequently the advice they really need, for they may strongly suspect the diagnosis in any case, and to deny them the information they require, because of timidity in giving them the diagnosis, deprives them of the essential part of the consultation.

Time may be necessary to overcome their resistance and more than one consultation may be required. A useful approach is to ask them to estimate the developmental age of their child before diagnostic testing, and frequently this coincides with the results of the test, showing that their awareness of the situation was more accurate than they would admit.

What advice should one give to mental defectives who wish to marry?

There has been considerable resistance on the part of society to permitting mental defectives to marry and this attitude has been based on a variety of factors, such as theories of inherited defects, inability to care for children, unbridled procreation and the extention of legal prohibitions concerning carnal knowledge of a certified defective. What is usually lacking is information on what does happen when mental defectives do marry. When such enquiries are undertaken, certain differences are evident between them and other members of the community. Family size is larger, infant mortality is higher; most men are able to work, criminality tends to be higher; broken marriages are commoner; and child care tends to be less effective.

On the other hand, temperamentally stable defective mothers can cope with their households fairly well when they have one or two children, but the family responsibilities outgrow their capacity and they become overwhelmed. What should still be done is to compare these families with families in the same social situation who are not defective rather than compare them with the rest of the community.

SECTION 18

PSYCHOLOGICAL AND PHYSICAL TREATMENTS

What does **psychotherapy** mean?

It is a technique usually based on a theory which is used in the treatment of psychological disorders. It is based on the establishment of a relationship between patient and therapist, and on the communications proceeding from the patient to the therapist, and vice versa. Interpretation of the material produced by the patient will depend on the theoretical construct by which the psychotherapist operates. Commoner forms of psychotherapy are psychoanalysis, analytical psychology, individual psychotherapy (based on the work of Alfred Adler), behaviour therapy, group psychotherapy, existential psychotherapy, psychodrama, hypnosis, and a variety of others which are not so well known.

Enumerate the essential factors in **psychoanalytic treatment**

These are:

(1) *The selection of the patient*, which is based on the following factors: (*a*) ego functioning, which means the capacity for reality testing; (*b*) strong motivation; (*c*) the capacity of the patient for psychological work; (*d*) the capacity of the patient and his family or the State to pay for what is essentially a very expensive treatment.

(2) *Free association*. This is the technique which is generally employed, and consists of the patient being put into a relaxed state and asked to allow whatever comes into his mind to be spoken while in a neutral and permissive setting.

(3) *Resistance*. This includes all those conscious and unconscious factors which interfere with a rational recovery-motivated ego. It need not be confined to the negative transference, which is a hostile attitude on the patient's part, for a very strong positive transference, which is the reverse, may prompt the patient to substitute love rather than experience the painful uncovering and understanding of unconscious guilt processes.

277

(4) *Transference*. This is generally referred to as positive feelings the patient has towards the analyst, but it also includes negative feelings and both these attitudes derive from earlier emotional relationships with other figures which have been transferred to the analyst. The neurotic and other inappropriate attitudes towards the analyst by the patient are referred to as *transference neurosis*. These help the analyst to gain insight into the patient's character structure. Interpretation is the analyst's efforts to try and correlate the patient's statements and attitudes with his unconscious mental functioning.

(5) *Counter-transference*. This is a transference reaction of the analyst to the patient and may prove a formidable obstacle to treatment should it get out of control.

The process of the treatment consists of a *working through*. The old resistances which have been dealt with may return and these have got to be repeatedly re-analysed.

(6) *Termination of treatment*. This is a matter for considerable debate and frequently it is the patient who feels sufficiently independent of the therapist who initiates this procedure.

There are many varieties of the treatment, but the orthodox methods consist of daily sessions of 50 minutes each with a minimum of five sessions a week, and the process may go on for three or more years. Modifications of the classical Freudian approach have been devised by a number of workers called the Neo-Freudians (for the theoretical basis of their work, see Section 2).

What is meant by **behaviour therapy**?

This is a form of psychotherapy based on Pavlovian principles and methods of treatment are by reciprocal inhibition, negative practice, aversion therapy and positive conditioning. The theory denies that there are unconscious factors in mental illness and regards neurosis not as a disease but as a collection of symptoms acquired as conditioned reflexes. The treatment is largely practised by non-medical psychologists who employ a model based on Hull's theory which expresses in mathematical terms the factors determining the formation and apparent extinction of conditioned reflexes. The treatment is claimed to be a highly scientific one, but this ignores the essential relationship which is established between therapist and patient as in all forms of psychotherapy. Where psychiatric illness has a large habit component, behaviour therapy has claimed good results and it is now being used for alcoholism, homosexuality and other sexual perversions, compulsive delinquent behaviour, gambling and even for the aggressive, thrusting car-driver. In these conditions and in phobic anxiety results compare favourably with individual and group psychotherapy.

It is growing in popularity in the treatment of phobic anxiety states. A hierarchical list of symptoms is prepared by the patient and progress is from the least-feared to the most-feared. Various techniques are employed such as reciprocal inhibition which creates a relaxed atmosphere, sometimes with the help of sedatives like intravenous barbiturates or minor tranquillisers like intravenous diazepam. Suggestion is employed and the patient encouraged to extend the range of activity till all fears are overcome. A 'token economy treatment' based on operant conditioning may also be employed. (See Section 1.)

Aversion measures such as electric shocks as a form of deconditioning or 'throwing the patient in at the deep end' (*implosion therapy*) are frequently used. The psychiatrist is not relieved of his responsibility to make an accurate formulation of the patient's problems and decide whether there are other areas of instability which may require an entirely different approach or whether the behaviour therapy techniques may in themselves be harmful. It is difficult if not impossible to delegate such functions to other professional workers such as psychologists and social workers and it is likely that the ethical and clinical place of such treatment in the hands of relatively unsupervised personnel will attract much attention and debate.

Write an essay on group psychotherapy

Society has, since prehistoric times, organised itself in groups for support of those in need and more specialised groups have throughout history banded themselves together for their own emotional well-being or the glory of God. Modern group psychotherapy as a branch of psychological medicine is relatively recent and depended on the formulation of group dynamics,

K

which were inspired by the two-body relationship of individual psychotherapy.

Theoretical considerations

In addition to Freudian psychopathology, group psychotherapy makes use of Le Bon's concept of the 'Group Mind' which stresses that a group differs from the individuals that compose it and possesses a sort of collective mind which makes it feel, think and act in a manner which is very different from its constituent parts. Members of a group lack inhibition and contact between one member of the group and the other is encouraged, so that feelings are rapidly transmitted through the group; they are also extremely suggestible. Groups are either *didactic* or *directive* where a leader takes charge and the others are prepared to follow, or as is mostly practised in this country, the group is *leaderless or non-directive*, and this method is favoured by the two pioneers in group therapy, Slavson in America and Foulkes in Britain. Selection of patients is most important as certain personality disorders tend to disrupt the group and others are unable to benefit by it. Similarly, the arrangement of the group may be important in that a retiring and sensitive person, when placed between two more active members, may be brought into the group situation but if placed on the outside he may be extruded. There has been tremendous enthusiasm for group psychotherapy, in Britain particularly, and elsewhere and many mental hospitals have organised their whole régime on a group therapy basis. It remains to be seen whether this is as effective as other less dynamic orientated therapies. Some attempts at validation have shown that some patients tend to stay in hospital much longer, or become addicted to the situation without really benefiting from it.

What is **existential psychiatry?**

This is a recent reaction against the rationalism and objectivity of the psychoanalytic movement and derives its inspiration from a similar reaction by Kierkegaard against the intellectualisation of the Church. A number of philosophers have been claimed by the movement, and these include Buber, Kierkegaard, Nietzsche, Sartre and Schopenhauer; authors and painters have also been claimed as the inspiration of the group. Existentialism seeks to characterise Man through its 'dynamic' formulations rather than through its 'essence'. This dynamic has been called *existence*.

It derives from the Protestant ideology of the I-Thou relationship which states that Man is continually seeking for his existence, and any attempt to help him without recognising this essential factor is unlikely to succeed.

It has developed a vocabulary of its own with the word *Dasein* (German for existence) equalling the verb, *being*. The process of treatment is called *Daseinanalyse*.

Write a short note on **psychodrama**

This is a technique of psychotherapy which derives from Moreno, who, in Vienna, introduced this method in his Theatre of Spontaneity which he founded in 1921. The ingredients are (1) the protagonist, or subject, (2) the director or chief therapist, (3) the auxiliary egos and (4) the group. The purpose of the treatment is to re-enact on the stage the patients' problems and a number of methods are used to overcome resistance such as allowing the patient to play the role of the patient, or caricaturising serious problems, or replacing the therapist by an auxiliary to meet the needs of the patient. This too, has developed its own jargon, and modifications of the treatment have been introduced such as hypnodrama, direct analysis, accessory drug therapy where stimulants such as caffeine, lysergic acid and methedrine have been used to stimulate the patient, didactic psychodrama where members of the staff may act the part of the patient or his relatives, rehearsed psychodrama where he writes his own play and other patients and staff rehearse their parts, and conditioned psychodrama which is based on Pavlovian principles. A traumatic situation which has resulted in distressing symptoms is re-enacted until the symptoms no longer occur. Further modifications are constantly being developed.

Give an account of **hypnosis**

Hypnosis is a form of psychotherapy which, in modern times, derives from the work and demonstrations of Anton Mesmer, a Viennese doctor who was popular in Paris before the Revolution. He claimed that it was based on animal magnetism, but this was later discounted and since then the London physician Elliotson gave it a more orthodox place in medical treatment. It was Charcot, with his demonstrations of hypnosis at the Salpêtrière in Paris, who made the method extremely popular in Europe and emphasised its value in the removal of hysterical symptoms.

The technique

This is essentially simple and requires very little training. It consists of the constant repetition of a suggestion to the patient of relaxation and/or sleep. When this has been effected, various suggestions are made to the patient in this state of trance, which are helpful either for the removal of symptoms or the elucidation of psychiatric problems by the recovery of earlier memories. Psychiatric *contraindications* are the hysterical character, the schizophrenic, paranoid states, psychotic depression and obsessional states. It acts best in hysterical symptoms, psychosomatic disorders, tics and habit spasms including stammering, particularly in children, in the production of anaesthesia for surgery and childbirth, analytical hypnotherapy and dermatology. The mode of action is still unknown.

What is meant by **superficial psychotherapy**?

There are a variety of forms. Most depend on the doctor-patient relationship which invests the doctor with healing powers and ascribes to him an authority which has a powerful influence on the patient. Suggestion is therefore facilitated, positive advice is accepted and placebos are given the force of potent drugs. If the doctor is gentle, he fills the patient's need for a comforting, maternal figure; a positive and authoritarian doctor may help the patient to accept him as a father figure. These superficial methods are frowned on by orthodox trained analysts, yet patients receive considerable benefit from such attentions. There are structured forms of such psychotherapy which consist of techniques of persuasion and are not far removed from some of those employed by behaviour therapists.

Write a short note on **brief psychotherapy**

A number of analysts were rather dissatisfied with the length of time required for orthodox psychoanalysis, and short-cut methods have been devised. It has been shown that in a number of patients such short-cut methods based on psychoanalytical concepts have effected considerable improvements. Malan has been able to validate the results in patients treated this way, showing that the results are as good as one would have expected had they been submitted to a much longer course of treatment. Similar claims have been made previously by Franz Alexander.

Describe the administration and effects of ECT (electroplexy)

This treatment consists of the passage of electric current through the forehead of the patient, one electrode being applied to each temple. The machines currently used supply a steady current of approximately 100 volts for 0·5 second. The patient is starved of food and drink for three to four hours prior to treatment and is asked to empty his bladder immediately before treatment. Before treatment begins it must be ensured that dentures are removed and that metallic objects are removed from the hair of the head.

ECT is now usually given in a modified form, i.e. the convulsion is modified by a muscle relaxant such as succinylcholine. The patient is pre-medicated with 0·6 mg. of atropine which can be given intravenously together with thiopentone or methylhexitone immediately before the muscle relaxant is administered. Atropine prevents cardiac arrhythmias due to vagal slowing and reduces secretions. Anaesthetic and relaxant drugs render the patient unconscious and apnoeic. He is given oxygen before the current is applied and a gag is placed between the teeth to prevent biting of the tongue or lips during the fit. At the completion of the tonic and clonic phases of the convulsion, which in unmodified cases resembles a grand mal epileptic fit, the patient is oxygenated until he resumes breathing on his own account. Two doctors should assist with treatment and one of them should have experience in anaesthesia and resuscitation.

ECT has both psychological and physical effects. (1) *Physical*: blood pressure is raised and temporary cardiac arrhythmias as well as autonomic effects on the heart rate and sphincters may be seen. (2) *Psychological*: immediately consciousness is regained following the fit there is a short period of confusion with amnesia, the latter sometimes persisting for several hours. Headaches and memory loss which last for days after ECT are almost always functional in origin. The tendency to amnesia and confusion is heightened in patients who have any cerebral disease, e.g. cerebral arteriosclerosis or early dementia.

What is **unilateral ECT?**

Various workers have found that, when unilateral ECT is applied to the non-dominant side of the skull, memory impairment seems less likely to develop later than with unilateral ECT to the dominant side or in the case of the more traditional bilateral ECT. Views on the therapeutic efficacy of unilateral ECT vary, and there have been suggestions that with unilateral ECT a greater number of treatments are necessary to achieve the same degree of recovery from severe depression. Furthermore, controlled trials with satisfactory tests for memory loss are difficult to organise and the determining of the non-dominant side is not without its problems.

How does **ECT** work?

This remains unclear. The early view that there was an inverse relationship between epilepsy and certain other mental disorders has not been substantiated. *Theories* of action include: (1) That its efficacy is due to the *amnesia* and that the patients thereby lose their symptoms. There is very little support for this contention. (2) *Biochemical*: many changes have been demonstrated in patients and animals following the administration of ECT including alterations in steroid and amine metabolism. It is likely that many of these effects are secondary and not specifically related to therapeutic effect. (3) *Neurophysiological*: there is evidence from animal experiments that changes are produced in the limbic system including the temporal lobes and it is known that the latter play some role in the emotional life. (4) A *computer* analogy suggests that ECT works by rectifying abnormal neuronal circuits which allegedly are associated with certain mental disorders. It is hypothesised that the effect of ECT is similar to that of the electric charge which normalises the abnormally functioning computer which has associated aberrant electrical circuits.

What are the **indications and contraindications** for ECT?

1. *Indications.* It is of greatest therapeutic value in cases of

psychotic depression and in catatonic stupor, and is also given, coupled with major tranquillisers, in mania and in early cases of schizophrenia. The number of treatments in any one course varies, but on average the treatment is given two to three times weekly up to a total of six to ten treatments, tailing off the last few on a weekly basis. In some acute emergencies such as depressive or catatonic stupor, ECT may have to be applied daily for several treatments.

2. *Contraindications.* (*a*) Anaesthetic risks. Patients who are old, frail or physically infirm, especially if there is associated cardiac failure are poor risks. Skeletal disease is no longer a contraindication since with modified ECT, i.e. employing anaesthetic and relaxant drugs, risk of fractures or dislocations is reduced to almost nil. Obvious anaesthetic risks include recent myocardial infarction and severe respiratory disease. (*b*) Organic brain disease. ECT tends to exacerbate many brain diseases, e.g. G.P.I., cerebral tumour, primary dementia, disseminated sclerosis, encephalopathies, and any state associated with clouding of consciousness. (*c*) Psychiatric. Neuroses tend to be made worse.

Describe some varieties of **prefrontal leucotomy (lobotomy)**

1. *The standard operation.* This consists of a bilateral division of the white fibres of the centrum ovale in a plane slightly anterior to the anterior horns of the lateral ventricles. The standard operation has largely been replaced by modified forms of the operation such as the following.

2. *Rostral leucotomy.* This consists of bilateral cutting of the fronto-thalamic fibres in the antero-medial quadrants of the frontal lobes. There are a number of variations of this technique.

3. *Cortica undercuttings.* This entails bilateral cutting of the white matter under areas 9 and 10, or 10 and 11 of the cerebral cortex.

4. *Transorbital.* This involves penetration of the orbital plate with severing of the fronto-thalamic fibres in the infero-medial quadrants.

5. *Stereotaxic.* This technique is similar to that used for operations for Parkinsonism. A lesion is placed in the dorso-medial nucleus of the thalamus by chemical or electrical coagula-

tion. Radio-active yttrium has been used to produce a lesion in the fronto-orbital region and reports have been encouraging. This method may be of value in elderly or arteriosclerotic subjects where surgery would be dangerous. Lesions have also been made in the limbic system (limbic leucotomy) or in the cingulate gyrus (cingulectomy).

6. *Ultrasonic methods.* Destruction of tissue employing irradiation techniques is the basis of this variety of leucotomy. Experience remains limited and mainly reserved for cases of intractable pain.

Describe the **effects of prefrontal leucotomy** *operations*

The operation tends to reduce anxiety and tension, especially in those with driving and obsessional types of personality. The intensity of the patient's affect tends to be diminished with consequent reduction in depression, especially in those of good previous personality. Disinhibition of behaviour is produced, the patient acquiring a less restrained pattern with relative unconcern.

Side-effects of the operation

1. *Immediate.* A period of confusion is not uncommon but tends to be short-lived, especially in a modified operation. In the standard operation there is also a risk of intra-cerebral bleeding. In fit patients there should not be any appreciable mortality, though it was 2 to 3 per cent with the standard operation. Post-operative aggressive behaviour is frequently seen, especially in those who, prior to operation, had difficulty in expressing their hostility, e.g. in obsessional neurotics.

2. *Remote.* Personality changes are common after leucotomy and in a mild form are desirable. Occasionally disinhibition of behaviour and emotional display may lead to light-hearted and objectionable conduct. These effects are far more common in operations associated with a more posterior cut and in patients who have been poorly selected for the operation. Permanent intellectual deficit is uncommon following a modified operation unless there has been some underlying brain disease, e.g. arterio-sclerosis or early dementia. Post-leucotomy epilepsy is un-common and is usually controllable with anti-convulsant drugs. A generalised apathy and loss of interest is seen especially in those

cases where there is poor family support and an inadequate programme of rehabilitation.

Comment on the indications for leucotomy

1. *Depression.* Patients who do well are in the middle and older age-groups with a good previous personality and whose depression has not responded satisfactorily to the conventional methods of treatment, or where there is increasingly frequent relapse. Recurrent neurotic depression does not do well and is a contra-indication. In many depressives the episodes of psychotic depression become more manageable by the previously ineffective treatment.

2. *Neuroses.* In obsessional neuroses and chronic anxiety states where the previous personality is that of an effective, driving conscientious individual with no tendency to drug addiction.

3. *Other conditions.* Leucotomy is occasionally performed in cases of intractable pain and in the past has been employed in the treatment of schizophrenia, but it is doubtful whether the latter illness constitutes a present-day indication. In recommending leucotomy, the following factors must be taken into consideration: (*a*) adequate selection of patients, (*b*) choosing the right operation for the particular patient, (*c*) early mobilisation and rehabilitation of the patient with mustering of family support. A lack of the latter constitutes a contraindication to the operation.

LEGAL PSYCHIATRY

With which patients does the **Mental Health Act** **(1959)** *deal?*

This Act states that patients may be admitted to psychiatric hospitals as 'informal patients', i.e. no formalities are necessary and the patients have the same status as any patients admitted to general hospitals. The Act deals with the following categories of patients: those suffering from *mental disorder.* This broad generic term includes mental illness, subnormality and psychopathic disorder. *Psychopathic disorder* is defined as a persistent disorder or disability of mind which results in abnormally aggressive or seriously irresponsible conduct on the part of the patient, and requires, or is susceptible to treatment. *Subnormality* means a state of arrested or incomplete development of the mind which includes subnormal intelligence and is of a nature or degree which requires, or is susceptible to treatment, or other special care or training of the patient. *Severe subnormality* means a state of arrested or incomplete development of mind which includes subnormal intelligence and is of such a nature or degree that the patient is incapable of living an independent life or guarding himself against exploitation.

What **Orders** *are commonly employed* **to detain** *a patient for (involuntary) psychiatric treatment?*

Section 25 is an Observation Order which lasts for 28 days and requires two medical signatures, one being by a psychiatrist approved under Section 28 of the Mental Health Act. In this Section it must be stated that the patient is suffering from mental disorder which warrants detention in hospital for observation, that he ought to be so detained for his own health or safety, or for the health or safety of others. *Section 26* is a Treatment Order for those suffering from mental disorder, for example, mental illness or severe subnormality at any age or psychopathy or mental subnormality for those under 21. The duration of the Treatment

Order is one year in the first instance, renewable every two years. It must be stated that the patient warrants detention for treatment, that this is necessary for his health or safety, or for the protection of others. Under these two Sections an interval not exceeding seven days is allowable to make a recommendation. *Section 29* is an Emergency Order which requires only one medical signature and this may be that of the family doctor; the duration is 72 hours. *Section 30* applies to those who are already in hospital, and allows the patient to be detained against his will for a period not exceeding three days. At the end of this period an Observation Order may be made, or the patient may revert to informal status. *Section 136* allows a constable to take anyone from a public place to a place of safety including a mental hospital; the duration of this Order is 72 hours.

Describe the commonly used Court Orders

Patients having committed minor offences not punishable by imprisonment are often dealt with after psychiatric assessment under Section 25 or 26. *Section 60* may be used by any Court, including a Magistrate's Court if, on the written or oral evidence of two doctors, one of whom must be approved under the Mental Health Act, that the patient, having committed an offence punishable by summary conviction with imprisonment, is suffering from mental disorder. Under Section 60 the Court sends the patient for psychiatric treatment and there is no imprisonment, no fine, and no probation. The responsible medical officer has the authority to discharge the patient when he deems it suitable. *Section 61* makes similar provision for children. *Section 65* is similar to Section 60 excepting that there is a restriction on discharge and the patient has usually committed a more serious crime, having appeared before a Crown Court. The patient is dischargeable only on the order of the Secretary of State. *Section 71* allows the Secretary of State to direct, through the Court, that the patient be detained during Her Majesty's pleasure if he is found to be insane at his trial. *Section 72* allows for the removal to a psychiatric hospital of someone who becomes mentally ill while serving a sentence of imprisonment. *Section 73* allows the detention for psychiatric assessment and treatment of persons suspected of being mentally ill who are in custody, or who have been remanded in custody, usually on order of a higher Court. Under *Section 4 of the Criminal Justice Act (1948)* patients may be referred for psychiatric treatment under probation order. In this way, part of their probation order is that they either attend an out-patient clinic or are admitted to hospital for a minimal specified period.

Comment on criminal responsibility

The question of criminal responsibility mainly arises in the context of major crime. In the case of less serious offences the mentally disordered are often dealt with under the provisions of one of the sections of the Mental Health Act (1959). In a major crime such as murder, a defence on the grounds of insanity has often been made. The McNaghten Rules enunciated in 1843 stated that to establish such a defence it must be clearly proved that, at the time of committing the act, the accused was labouring under some mental disorder, such that he did not know the nature of the act, or if he did know, he did not know that what he was doing was wrong. Extension of knowledge in psychiatry has helped to render these rules obsolete.

The Homicide Act (1957) brought in the principle of diminished responsibility in certain types of murder, thus medico-legal arguments about insanity are now less likely to take place. A verdict of manslaughter can be substituted for murder where it is shown that the accused was suffering from some degree of mental disturbance which substantially impaired his mental responsibility for his behaviour. This Act also reduces the offence of the survivor of a suicide pact to one of manslaughter.

An individual cannot be tried unless he is fit to defend himself. In a higher Court a claim may be made that the offender is *unfit to plead*, either at the beginning of the trial (on arraignment), or during the trial itself. Certain *criteria* of fitness to plead are laid down: (1) The prisoner should be able to instruct his Counsel. (2) He should appreciate the significance of pleading 'Guilty' or 'Not Guilty'. (3) He should be able to challenge a juror. (4) He should be able to examine witnesses. (5) He should be able to understand and follow the evidence placed before the Court, and Court procedure. In practice, unfitness to plead is often established when the prisoner is being medically assessed in prison.

The commonest psychiatric causes are mental subnormality, schizophrenia and occasionally organic states. In cases of major crime the accused, having been found unfit to plead, has in the past been detained 'until Her Majesty's pleasure be known' in a special (Broadmoor) type of hospital. Under the Criminal Procedure (Insanity) Act (1964), a verdict of Not Guilty by reason of insanity is substituted for the old verdict of Guilty but Insane. The latter verdict used to lead to detention during Her Majesty's pleasure. This Act allows such mentally ill offenders and those found unfit to plead to be dealt with under the provisions of the Mental Health Act (1959). It also provides for those found unfit to plead to be remanded for psychiatric reports, and treatment if necessary, with subsequent appearance at a trial when they are mentally fit.

What is meant by **testamentary capacity?**

This is the capacity of a person to make a will, and it usually rests on the following: (1) The individual must know the nature and extent of his property. (2) He must be cognisant of the persons who have a natural claim on his bounty. (3) His judgment must be so unclouded as to enable him to evaluate the relative strength of these claims. (4) The testator must appreciate the nature and effect of his act. (5) He must be of full age and of sound disposing mind. Sound disposing mind does not necessarily mean that the subject must not be suffering from any illness, for it is possible for someone who is the subject of a major mental disorder to be capable of making a valid will. The commonest problem in testamentary capacity is that of a senile patient who has difficulties with his memory and may, or may not, have delusions.

In doubtful cases the problem can be avoided by appointing a receiver. The Court of Protection exists to manage the property and affairs of persons who by reason of mental disorder are unable to do so themselves. It acts by appointing a receiver.

What are the psychiatric implications of **the Matrimonial Causes Act** (*1965*)?

In the terms of this Act, a marriage may be declared void on the grounds that, at the time of marriage, either party (1) was of unsound mind or (2) was suffering from mental disorder within the meaning of the Mental Health Act (1959) of such a kind or to such an extent as to be unfitted for marriage and the procreation of children or (3) was subject to recurrent attacks of insanity or epilepsy.

Each of these criteria are open to wide interpretation. Legal battles have been fought in the courts in attempts to declare marriages void where one of the partners has been subject to episodes of psychiatric illness. For instance, there have been cases where a husband has petitioned for his marriage to be deemed void because his wife has been admitted to hospital on several occasions for psychiatric reasons. Admission of itself does not satisfy any of the above criteria. In a celebrated judgment in 1969 (Bennett *v.* Bennett), several admissions for 'hysterical neurosis' on the part of the wife were not regarded as sufficient grounds under this Act, and the husband's petition was dismissed. It is also very difficult to invoke (1) above, unless the spouse has persisted in his/her mental illness, which usually needs to be psychotic in nature.

'Unfitted for marriage' on account of mental disorder within the meaning of the Mental Health Act (1959) has been equated with an inability to fulfil the obligations of normal married life, and to conduct a normal life generally. Psychotic illness, psychopathic disorder or subnormality could on occasions qualify.

Comment on the relationship between **mental illness and delinquency**

The majority of those members of the population who indulge in delinquent behaviour are not mentally ill. Many offenders, especially those who habitually are convicted, tend to have psychopathic personalities rather than be subject to any mental illness. Psychopaths constitute a high proportion of chronic recidivists. Of persistent criminals in prison about 20 per cent are either mentally ill, or have been mentally ill in the past. (1) Personality disorders: psychopaths frequently offend against the law and may be subject to aggressive, impulsive behaviour. Sexual deviants frequently come into conflict with the law. Severe personality disorder is often the background to the development of drug addiction, which in itself may lead to conviction on account of stealing, forged prescriptions, possession of dangerous drugs, etc. (2) Schizophrenia: these patients, especially in the chronic stages of their illness may indulge in petty offences mainly involving theft, or damage to property, seldom offending the person. Schizophrenics sometimes deteriorate to vagrancy with its frequently associated conflicts with the law. Simple schizophrenia sometimes leads to a psychopathic type of personality deterioration and may become associated with petty crime or drug addiction. (3) Organic psychiatric disorders: these may be associated with disinhibited, and therefore anti-social, conduct and the first manifestation of frontal lobe disease or dementia may be delinquent behaviour. The man who is beginning to dement may expose himself in public. (4) Epilepsy: this may be associated with states of so-called 'automatism' or other states of altered consciousness. It is unusual for crime to be committed during such states, however. Epileptics are often sensitive to alcoholic excesses and this may lead them into trouble. There are rare cases reported of temporal lobe lesions being associated with crime or sexual perversion. (5) Affective disorder: the manic patient may lack propriety in his business or social conduct which may lead him into conflict with the law, e.g. he may, on account of grandiose thinking, involve himself in large-scale financial transactions. Depression, if sufficiently severe, may lead to an attempt at suicide; since the 1961 Suicide Act this is no longer an offence. Rarely, the patient subject to psychotic depression may decide to commit suicide but not before murdering those close to him in an attempt to relieve them of their supposed misery and doom. Middle-aged women charged with shoplifting occasionally have a mild agitated type of depression. (6) Subnormality: mentally defective individuals often lack social decorum and act irresponsibly; this may lead to petty crime or promiscuity.

Discuss **termination of pregnancy on psychiatric grounds**

In recent years, changing social attitudes and values have become reflected in new legislation on homosexuality, divorce, suicide, homicide and abortion.

Under the Abortion Act (1967), termination of pregnancy is legalised on four grounds:

1. The continuance of the pregnancy would involve risk to the life of the pregnant woman greater than if the pregnancy were terminated.

2. The continuance of the pregnancy would involve risk of injury to the physical or mental health of the pregnant woman greater than if the pregnancy were terminated.

3. The continuance of the pregnancy would involve risk of injury to the physical or mental health of the existing child or children of the family of the pregnant woman greater than if the pregnancy were terminated.

4. There is a substantial risk that if the child were born it would suffer from such physical or mental abnormalities as to be seriously handicapped.

Before a therapeutic abortion is performed, a certificate must be signed by two registered medical practitioners, indicating which of the aforementioned criteria are being invoked. There is no reference in the Act to the effect that, where psychiatric or social factors are the indications, a psychiatrist should be one of the signatories, and neither need the person performing the operation be a signatory.

In cases where the so-called 'social clause' is being considered, viz. possible future effects on the existing children, an intimate knowledge of the family background and circumstances is essential; and the family doctor is more appropriate in this respect than a specialist.

The psychiatrist's expertise is called for in giving an opinion on the advisability of abortion on grounds that continuation of the pregnancy would involve risk to the mental health of the pregnant woman. There are very few, if any, psychiatric indications for termination, though chronic schizophrenia and severe subnormality have been considered by some to constitute such indications. There is no reliable evidence that neurotic illness is aggravated materially by pregnancy and many actually improve, though after childbirth the neurotic handicap may reassert.

Although pregnant women with depressive illnesses and reactions are frequently referred for an opinion on the advisability of termination, such conditions are nearly always treatable or transient. Some of these reactions are in the nature of situational stress reactions following the woman's knowledge of her pregnant state. Suicide is extremely rare in pregnant women.

Opinion varies to a large extent among doctors as to the weight given to social factors in arriving at a decision on therapeutic abortion.

Psychiatric sequelae to therapeutic abortion are not infrequent, the commonest being a depressive syndrome with feelings of guilt. Severe psychiatric illness may follow abortion and usually occurs in women with a history of mental illness. It is perhaps paradoxical that those in whom psychiatric indications for termination can be found are most liable to psychiatric complications of therapeutic abortion and the psychiatrist's role under the new Act is to advise his colleagues when not to abort.

Further reading

It has been the policy of *Basic Psychiatry* not to burden the readers with references, for this would detract from its usefulness as a means to rapid revision or as a simple introductory text. If more detailed information is required with access to a large and comprehensive bibliography, the reader should consult *Guide to Psychiatry* by Myre Sim which is also published by Churchill Livingstone.

INDEX